Judith M. Wilkinson, PhD, ARNP

Leslie S. Treas, PhD, RN, CPNP-PC, NNP-BC

POCKET
Nursing Skills
What You Need to Know Now

 F.A. Davis Company • Philadelphia

Purchase additional copies of this book at your health science bookstore or directly from F.A. Davis by shopping online at www.fadavis.com or by calling 800-323-3555 (US) or 800-665-1148 (CAN)

F. A. Davis Company
1915 Arch Street
Philadelphia, PA 19103
www.fadavis.com

Printed in China

Last digit indicates print number: 10 9 8 7 6 5 4 3 2 1

Publisher, Nursing: Lisa B. Houck
Director of Content Development: Darlene D. Pedersen
Senior Project Editor: Meghan K. Ziegler
Cover Design: Carolyn O'Brien

Tabs & Table of Contents

Tab 9 - IV Infusions 112

Tab 10 - Nutrition 146

Tab 11 - Urinary 168

Tab 12 - Bowel 187

Tab 13 - Activity & Exercise 205

Tab 14 - Wound Healing 219

Universal Steps for All Procedures

These guidelines apply to every procedure in this handbook.

Note: All procedures are "rules of thumb." Everything you learn can be altered by medical orders, new information, agency policies, and individual patient needs. Every procedure requires nursing judgment.

Before Approaching the Patient

- Check medication records or obtain a prescription, if necessary.
- Follow agency protocols.
- Obtain a signed, informed consent, if needed.
- Wash your hands; don procedure gloves, if needed.
- Gather necessary supplies and equipment.
- Obtain assistance, if needed (e.g., to move a patient).

Prepare the Patient

- Introduce yourself, and any assistants, to the patient.
- Identify the patient: Read the wristband and ask the patient to state his name.
- Make relevant assessments to ensure that the patient still requires the procedure and can tolerate it, and that there are no contraindications.
- Explain the procedure to the patient, including what he will feel and need to do (e.g., "You will need to lie very still.").
- Provide privacy (e.g., ask visitors to step out, drape the patient).
- Use good body mechanics; position bed or treatment table to a working level; lower the near siderail.

During the Procedure

- Wash hands before touching the patient, before gloving, and after removing gloves.
- Observe universal precautions (e.g., don and change gloves when needed).
- Maintain sterility when needed.
- Maintain correct body mechanics.

■ Provide patient safety (e.g., keep siderail up on far side of the bed).
■ Continue to observe the patient while performing the procedure steps
and pause or stop the procedure if the patient is not tolerating it.
■ Follow correct procedure steps.

After the Procedure

■ Evaluate the patient's response to the procedure.
■ Leave the patient in a comfortable, safe position with the call light
within reach.
■ Return the bed to low position and raise the siderail (if appropriate).
■ Dispose of supplies and materials according to agency policy.
■ Wash hands again before leaving the room.
■ Document that the procedure was done; document patient responses.

Wilkinson Procedure 10-1. Admitting a Patient to Nursing Unit

✔️ For steps to follow in all procedures, refer to the first page of this book, Universal Steps for All Procedures.

Equipment
- Identifying wristband.
- Chart.
- Nursing admission database.
- Thermometer.
- BP cuff.
- Stethoscope.
- Scales.
- Patient gown.
- Admission pack (bath basin, pitcher, soap, comb, toothbrush, etc.).

Key Points
- Introduce yourself, assist the patient into a hospital gown, weigh, assist him into the bed.
- Be Smart! Allow extra time if patient is an older adult.
- Be Smart! Validate patient identity.
- Obtain a translator, if needed.
- Complete the nursing assessment, including VS; validate the admission list of medications.
- Provide information on:
  - Room.
  - Equipment.
  - Routines.
  - Nurse call system.
  - Advance directives.
  - Health Insurance Portability and Accountability Act (HIPAA).
- Answer any questions and provide printed information.
- Complete nursing admission forms according to agency policy.
- Complete or ensure that admission orders have been completed.

- Inventory the patient belongings; send home or lock up valuables.
- Finish the admission process: Ensure patient comfort (water, position-ing, pain).
- **Be Safe!** Make one last safety check: call light, bed position, siderails; and ask: "Is there anything else I can do for you?"
- **Be Safe!** Post "special needs" alerts for other caregivers (e.g., NPO, I&O).

Documentation

- Complete the admission database and nursing notes as needed.

Wilkinson Procedure 10-4. Discharging a Patient From Healthcare Facility

For steps to follow in all procedures, refer to the first page of this book, Universal Steps for All Procedures.

Equipment
- Medical record.
- Discharge form with patient instructions.
- Supplies for ongoing treatments.
- Patient's medications, clothes, personal care articles, and other belongings.
- Utility cart.
- Wheelchair.

Assessment
- Make a final, brief focused assessment, including:
  - Mobility.
  - Emotional and physical distress.
  - Ability to communicate and understand.

Key Points
Day or Two Days Before Discharge
- Arrange for or confirm transportation, and services and equipment needed at home. Also make necessary referrals.
- Teach patient/family about: patient's condition and medications, and how to use necessary equipment.
- Ask caregiver/family to bring clothing for patient to wear home.

Day of Discharge
- Perform and document final assessments.
- Be Safe! Confirm that patient has house keys, heat is turned on, and food is available.
- Make final notifications (e.g., transportation, community agencies).
- Pack patient's personal items and treatment supplies.
- Be Safe! Label take-home medications before giving to the patient.
- Provide prescriptions, instruction sheets, and appointment cards.
- Be Safe! Review discharge instructions with patient/family—especially regarding "high-risk" drugs such as anticoagulants, antibiotics, and sedatives.

- Answer any questions.
- Document final nursing note and complete the discharge summary.
- Accompany the patient out of the institution.
- Notify admissions department of the discharge.
- Ensure records are sent to the medical records department.

Documentation

- Complete the admission database and nursing notes.

Wilkinson Procedure 17-1. Assessing Body Temperature

✔️ For steps to follow in all procedures, refer to the first page of this book, Universal Steps for All Procedures.

Equipment

- Thermometer (generally, blue tip indicates oral and red tip indicates rectal) and cover.
- Tissues.
- Add as needed:
  - **Rectal:** Procedure gloves and water-soluble lubricant.
  - **Axillary:** Towel.
- Be Safe! Do not use a glass-and-mercury thermometer.

Assessment

- Assess for signs and symptoms of temperature alterations (e.g., diaphoresis).
- Assess for contraindications to the chosen site:
  - **Oral:** Do not use oral route for patients who cannot hold the thermometer properly, children, or those who use mouth breathing. If the patient has smoked, eaten, had a drink, or chewed gum, wait 20 to 30 minutes before taking oral temperature.
  - **Tympanic:** Assess for impacted earwax or hearing aid.
  - **Rectal:** Check the patient record for diarrhea or impacted stool.
  - **Axillary:** Check the record for presence of fever or hypothermia.
  - **Skin:** Assess for conditions that require an accurate, reliable reading (e.g., fever, hypothermia).

Key Points

- If the thermometer is not disposable, clean it before and after using.
- Select the appropriate site and thermometer, considering comfort, safety, and accuracy.
- Turn on, or otherwise ready the thermometer.
- Insert the thermometer in its sheath, or use a thermometer designated only for the patient.

- Insert. Leave an electronic thermometer in place until it beeps; for other thermometers use the recommended times.
  - **Glass thermometer:** Read at eye level after 5 to 8 minutes.
  - **Rectal site:** Read at eye level after 3 to 5 minutes.
- **Be Safe!** Do not use an oral thermometer to take a rectal temperature. Hold a rectal thermometer securely in place, and never leave it unattended.
  - **Axillary site:** Dry the axilla before inserting the thermometer.
  - **Tympanic site:** Refer to figures below for placement.
- Cleanse and store in recharging base (store glass thermometers safely to prevent breakage).

Documentation
- You will usually record temperature on a graphic or flowsheet.
- If you need to write a nursing note (e.g., because of a fever), notify the primary provider of the abnormal findings, and document according to agency policy:
  - Temperature, indicating the route of measurement.
  - Supporting findings, such as "Skin is hot and dry," and whether the temperature reading is consistent with the patient's condition.
  - Note previous recordings, if any.
- When evaluating, compare to normal range for developmental stage, site used, and patient's baseline data. Look for trends to identify potential concerns.

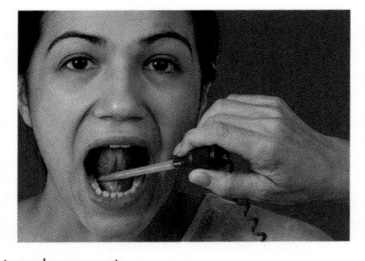

Oral thermometer placement.

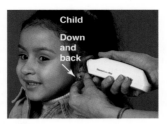

Tympanic thermometer: For a child, pull the pinna down and back.

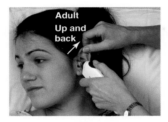

Tympanic thermometer: For an adult, pull the pinna up and back.

Wilkinson Procedure 17-2A. Assessing Radial Pulse

✅ For steps to follow in all procedures, refer to the first page of this book, Universal Steps for All Procedures.

Equipment
- Watch with a second hand or digital readout.
- Pen.
- Pencil.
- Flowsheet or personal digital assistant.

Assessment
- Determine why assessment of pulses is indicated.
- Assess factors that may alter the pulse, such as activity and medications.
- Be Smart! If the client has been recently active, wait 5 to 10 minutes before measuring.
- Be Smart! When analyzing findings, compare pulses bilaterally.

Post-Procedure Reassessment
- Be Safe! If pulse is not normal, observe for other indications of inadequate circulation, such as cool skin, decreased capillary refill, and bluish or ashen skin tone.
- Complete absence of pulse requires immediate intervention.

Key Points
- Make sure the client is resting while you assess the pulse.
- With client sitting or supine, flex the client's arm, and place the client's forearm across his chest.
- Palpate the radial artery.
- Place the pads of your index or middle fingers (or both) in the groove on the thumb side of the client's wrist, over the radial artery.
- Press lightly but firmly until you are able to feel the radial pulse. Start with light pressure to prevent occluding the pulse, and gradually increase the pressure until you feel the pulse well.
- Note the pulse rhythm (regular, irregular). Compare bilaterally.
- Note the quality of the pulse (bounding, strong, weak, or thready). Compare bilaterally.

- ■ **Be Smart!** Count the pulse. The first time you take the client's pulse, count for 60 seconds. After that:
  - ■ **For a regular pulse:** Count for 15 or 30 seconds and multiply by 4 or 2, respectively.
  - ■ **For an irregular pulse:** Count for 60 seconds.
- ■ Begin timing with the count of 1—the first beat that you feel.
- ■ For an admission assessment or peripheral vascular check, palpate the radial pulses on both wrists simultaneously.
- ■ For pedal, femoral, or temporal pulses, refer to the photos at the end of this procedure.

Documentation

- ■ Usually you will document the pulse rate on a flowsheet or graphic.
- ■ If you record it in a nursing note, document the rate, rhythm, quality, and site (e.g., "radial pulse 64 beats/min, regular, and strong bilaterally.")
- ■ Provide supporting evidence (e.g., "cool, pale skin") if you chart that pulses are decreased or absent.

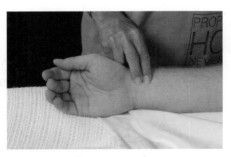

Radial pulse.

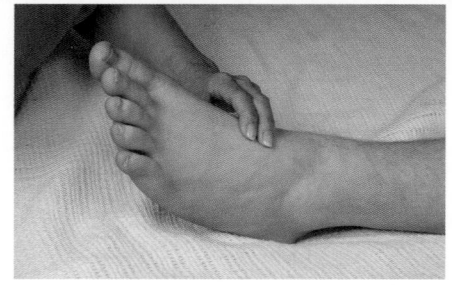

Pedal pulse.

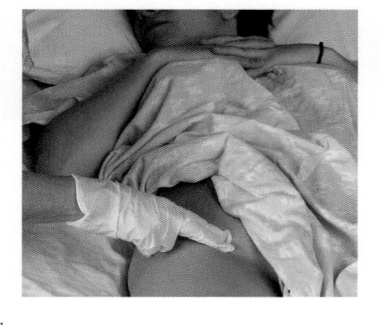

Femoral pulse.

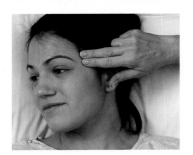

Temporal pulse.

Wilkinson Procedure 17-3. Assessing the Apical Pulse

✅ For steps to follow in all procedures, refer to the first page of this book, Universal Steps for All Procedures.

Equipment
- Watch with a second hand or digital readout.
- Stethoscope.
- Alcohol wipes.

Assessment
- Determine why assessment of the apical pulse is indicated.
- Assess factors that may alter the pulse, such as activity and medications.
- **Be Smart!** If the client has been recently active, wait 10 to 15 minutes before obtaining measurement.

Key Points
- Position client sitting, if possible, or supine if not.
- Palpate and place stethoscope at the 5th intercostal space in the midclavicular line (PMI, the apex).
- Count for 60 seconds.
- Note pulse rate, rhythm, and quality, and the S_1 and S_2 heart sounds.

Documentation
- Note and document:
  - Pulse rate, rhythm, and site.
  - Data and other factors supporting your findings (e.g., skin color).
  - Trends over time.
- **Be Safe!** Note whether findings are within normal limits. If not, note other factors supporting the findings; notify the primary care provider.

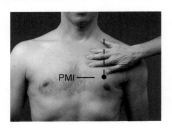

PMI

Apical pulse.

Wilkinson Procedure 17-4. Assessing an Apical–Radial Pulse Deficit

For steps to follow in all procedures, refer to the first page of this book, Universal Steps for All Procedures.

Equipment
- Watch or clock with a second hand or digital readout.
- Procedure gloves, if indicated.
- Stethoscope.
- Alcohol wipes.

Assessment
- Determine why assessment of pulse deficit is indicated (e.g., digitalis therapy, blood loss, cardiac or respiratory disease).
- Assess factors that may alter the pulse (e.g., activity and medications).

Post-Procedure Reassessment
- Be Safe! Look for trends.
- The presence of any apical–radial pulse deficit is abnormal.

Key Points
- Palpate and place the stethoscope over the apex of the heart (5th intercostal space in the midclavicular line).
- Palpate the radial pulse.
- Have two nurses carry out the procedure, if possible—one counting radial and one counting apical pulse.
- Count for 60 seconds, simultaneously.
- Compare the pulse rate at both sites; calculate the difference.

Documentation
- Note and document:
  - The apical–radial pulse deficit (compare to previous findings).
  - Other measures of cardiopulmonary status (e.g., skin color) to identify a decline in the patient's condition.

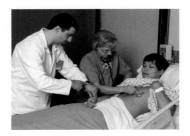

Assessing the apical–radial pulse deficit.

Wilkinson Procedure 17-5. Assessing Respirations

☑ For steps to follow in all procedures, refer to the first page of this book, Universal Steps for All Procedures.

Equipment
- A watch or clock with a second hand or digital readout.

Assessment
- Observe for signs of respiratory distress: breathing faster or slower than normal, gasping breaths, confusion, circumoral cyanosis.
- Determine the baseline respiratory rate and character of respirations.
- Assess for factors that may affect the respiratory rate (e.g., pain, activity, fever, respiratory disorders).

Key Points
- Count unobtrusively (e.g., while palpating the radial pulse).
- Count for 30 seconds if respirations are regular; for 60 seconds if they are irregular. A 60-second count is recommended for increased accuracy, even for regular respirations.
- Observe the rate, rhythm, and depth of respirations.

Evaluation and Documentation
- Usually, you will document routine VS (including respirations) on a graphic or flowsheet.
- When a nursing note is needed, document:
  - Respiratory rate and rhythm.
  - That respirations are either labored or unlabored.
  - If labored, describe in what way (e.g., intercostal retractions, use of accessory muscles, nasal flaring.)
- Be Smart! Compare to baseline findings. Note other VS, especially temperature. Look for trends. If respirations are not within normal limits, assess oxygenation with a pulse oximeter.

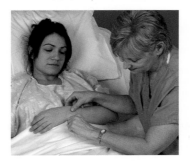

Assess respirations unobtrusively while palpating the pulse.

Wilkinson Procedure 17-6A. Measuring Blood Pressure in the Forearm

✔️ For steps to follow in all procedures, refer to the first page of this book, Universal Steps for All Procedures.

Equipment
- Stethoscope.
- 70% alcohol or benzalkonium chloride wipes.
- Sphygmomanometer with a cuff of the appropriate size.

Assessment
- Check for factors that can alter the readings (e.g., caffeine, smoking, exercise, stress).
- In determining which extremity to use, consider factors that affect circulation to the extremity and alter the reading (e.g., avoid an arm with an arteriovenous fistula, a deep vein thrombosis, a graft, schemic changes, an infusing IV, or on the side of a radical mastectomy).

Post-Procedure Reassessment
- Be Smart! When evaluating, check the previous recordings, if any.
- Because BP changes constantly and because so many factors affect it, you cannot draw conclusions from a single measurement.

Key Points
- If possible, place the patient in a sitting position, with the feet on the floor and the legs uncrossed.
- Measure BP after the patient has been inactive for 5 minutes (30 minutes, after strenuous exercise).
- Support the patient's arm at the level of the heart.
- Use a cuff of the appropriate size.
- Wrap the cuff snugly.
- Inflate the cuff while palpating the artery. Inflate to 30 mm Hg above the point at which you can no longer feel the artery pulsating.
- Place the stethoscope on the artery, and release pressure at 2 to 3 mm Hg per second.
- Record systolic/diastolic pressures (first and last sounds heard—e.g., 110/80 mm Hg).
- Be Smart! If you must remeasure, wait at least 2 minutes.

Documentation

- You will usually document BP on a flowsheet. If you chose an alternate site, document the site used and the reason for not using the upper arm.
  - Document the systolic/diastolic readings (e.g., 130/80 mm Hg).
  - *If you hear the 4th Korotkoff sound or muffling,* document systolic/muffling/diastolic (e.g., 130/80/70 mm Hg).
  - *If you hear an auscultatory gap,* document, for example "170/90 mm Hg with an auscultatory gap from 170 to 140 mm Hg."
  - Follow agency policy regarding the recording of muffled sounds.

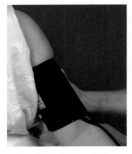

Wrap cuff snugly. Place about 1 in. (2.5 cm) above antecubital space.

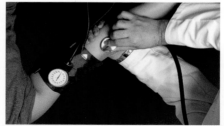

Place the stethoscope over the brachial artery.

Physical Exam

Wilkinson Procedure 19-20. Brief Bedside Assessment

✔️ For steps to follow in all procedures, refer to the first page of this book, Universal Steps for All Procedures.

Equipment
- Thermometer.
- Stethoscope.
- Sphygmomanometer.
- Procedure gloves.

Assessment
- Ask about any health problems, allergies, or medications.
- Ask your patient how he feels now and during the previous month and year.
- Ask other questions as you assess each body system.

Key Points
- Modify the procedure to fit the patient's health status.
- Observe the environment and the patient's general appearance.
- Measure VS, pain status, and pulse oximetry.
- Use a systematic (e.g., head-to-toe) approach.
- Assess the integument throughout the exam.
- Assess the head and neck.
- Assess the back with patient sitting.
- Assess the anterior chest (heart and lungs).
- Assess the abdomen with patient supine.
- Assess urinary status.
- Assess upper extremities, including edema and capillary refill.
- Assess lower extremities, including edema and capillary refill.
- Assess for spinal deformities with patient standing.
- Assess balance, coordination, ROM, and gait.
- While conducting the assessment and interacting with the patient, determine the patient's orientation to person, place, and time as well as appropriateness to situation.
- Check Babinski's reflex and Homans' sign.

Documentation

- Document your findings and report any significant changes or findings to the primary care provider.
- As a student, report your findings to the instructor and the patient's assigned RN for validation and action.

Wilkinson Procedure 20-1A. Hand Hygiene (Using Soap and Water)

✔️ For steps to follow in all procedures, refer to the first page of this book, Universal Steps for All Procedures.

Equipment
- Liquid soap (antimicrobial).
- Paper towels.
- Warm, running water.
- Hand moisturizer (optional).

Assessment
- Inspect the condition of your nails (no longer than ¼ in. from the fingertips, preferably no polish, definitely no chipped polish or artificial nails).
- Be Safe! Check your hands for breaks in the skin.

Key Points
- Remove your jewelry and watch.
- Wet your hands and wrists under running water.
- Apply 3 to 5 mL of liquid soap (or 3 to 4 pumps from a dispenser).
- Vigorously wash hands and fingers with warm water for at least 15 seconds (as long as it takes to sing *Happy Birthday*), lathering all surfaces.
- Clean under your fingernails.
- Rinse and dry your hands thoroughly.
- Turn off the faucet with a dry paper towel.

Documentation
- Hand hygiene is a responsibility of all healthcare providers. It does not require documentation.

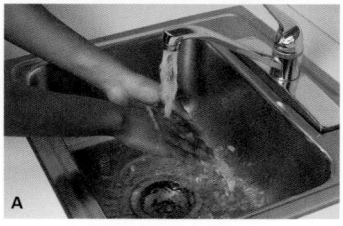

Keep your hands lower than your forearms.

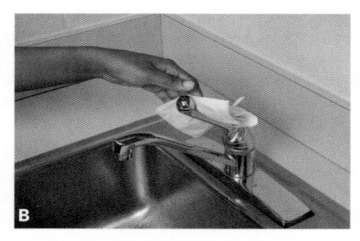

Use a dry paper towel to turn off the faucet.

Wilkinson Procedure 20-1B. Hand Hygiene (Using Alcohol-Based Handrubs)

☑ For steps to follow in all procedures, refer to the first page of this book, Universal Steps for All Procedures.

Equipment
- Alcohol-based handrub.
- Hand moisturizer (optional).

Assessment
- Inspect the condition of your nails (no longer than ¼ in. from the fingertips, preferably no polish, definitely no chipped polish or artificial nails).
- Be Safe! Check your hands for breaks in the skin.

Key Points
- Be Safe! Use alcohol-based handrubs when hands are not visibly soiled and when certain pathogens are suspected.
- Bare your hands and forearms. Push your sleeves above your wrists. Remove your jewelry and wristwatch.
- Apply a sufficient quantity (at least 3 mL) of the handrub solution to cover the hands and wrists.
- Vigorously rub the solution into the hands and fingers for 15 to 30 seconds (or as long as it takes to sing *Happy Birthday*), interlacing fingers, rubbing around each finger and thumb, including under the nails; and rubbing the backs and palms of the hands in a circular motion until the solution is completely dry.

Documentation
- Hand hygiene is a responsibility of all healthcare providers. It does not require documentation.

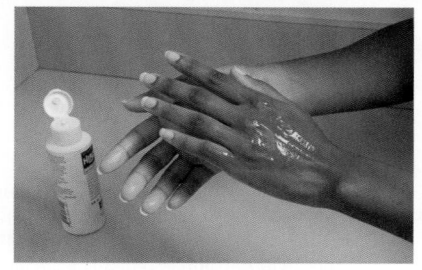

Rub vigorously, covering all surfaces of the hand and fingers.

Wilkinson Procedure 20-2. Donning Personal Protective Equipment

☑ For steps to follow in all procedures, refer to the first page of this book, Universal Steps for All Procedures.

Equipment

■ Following CDC recommendations, you will usually use some combination of these items, depending on the organism and level of precaution (e.g., you will use hair covers and shoe covers when full barrier precautions are needed):
  ■ Disposable gloves of the proper size.
  ■ Disposable isolation gown.
  ■ Face mask (or N-95 respirator mask, as indicated).
  ■ Face shield or goggles.
  ■ Hair cover.
  ■ Shoe covers.

Key Points

■ Be Safe! Before exposure, don appropriate PPE according to standard precautions or transmission guidelines.
■ The CDC sequence for donning PPE is:
  ■ First put on gown.
  ■ Apply a surgical mask for droplet isolation or an N-95 respirator mask for airborne isolation.
  ■ Put on goggles or a face shield.
  ■ Don gloves.

Documentation

■ The use of PPE is assumed and does not require documentation.

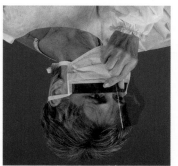

The mask must fit snugly to the face.

Wilkinson Procedure 20-3. Removing Personal Protective Equipment

✅ For steps to follow in all procedures, refer to the first page of this book, Universal Steps for All Procedures.

Equipment

- Following CDC recommendations, and depending on the organism and level of precaution, you will usually be wearing some combination of:
  - Gloves.
  - Gown.
  - Mask.
  - Eye protection.
- In certain situations, you may be wearing:
  - Hair covers.
  - Shoe covers (e.g., when full barrier precautions are needed).

Key Points

- **Be Safe!** Remove the PPE at the doorway before leaving the patient's room, or in an anteroom.
- **Be Safe!** Avoid contaminating self, others, or the environment when removing equipment.
- Considered contaminated: front areas, sleeves, mask, and gloves of the PPE (as well as head and shoe covers if you are wearing them).
- Considered clean: the inside of the gown, gloves, the ties on the mask, and ties at the back of the gown (as well as the inside of the head and shoe covers if you are wearing them).
- The CDC sequence for removing PPEs is:
  - Always remove gloves first.
  - Then take off the face shield or goggles.
  - Take off the gown next.
  - Remove the mask or respirator.
  - [The CDC does not specify, but if wearing shoe covers, remove them last.]
- Perform hand hygiene before leaving the room.

Documentation

- Removal of PPE is assumed and does not require documentation.

Wilkinson Procedure 20-4. Surgical Hand Washing: Traditional Method

☑ For steps to follow in all procedures, refer to the first page of this book, Universal Steps for All Procedures.

Equipment
- Antimicrobial soap (60% to 95% alcohol, or other FDA-approved for surgical hand asepsis).
- Soft, nonabrasive scrub sponge.
- Disposable single-use nail cleaner.
- Deep sink with foot or knee controls.
- Surgical shoe covers, cap, and face mask.
- Sterile gloves of the correct size.
- Surgical pack containing a sterile towel.

Key Points
- Don surgical shoe covers, cap, and face mask before the scrub.
- Use warm water.
- Perform a prewash, using soap and water.
- Clean under your nails under running water.
- Wet the scrub sponge, and apply a generous amount of antimicrobial soap.
- Using a circular motion, scrub all surfaces of nails, hands, and forearms at least 10 times, or the length of time specified by agency policy.
- Rinse hands and arms, keeping fingertips higher than your elbows.
- Grasp a sterile towel, and back away from the sterile field.
- Thoroughly dry your hands before donning sterile gloves.

Documentation
- A surgical hand scrub does not require documentation. In some agencies, you may record it on a checklist.

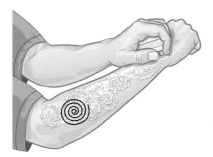

Use a circular motion. Keep hands higher than elbows.

Wilkinson Procedure 20-5. Surgical Hand Washing: Brushless System

✔️ For steps to follow in all procedures, refer to the first page of this book, Universal Steps for All Procedures.

Equipment
■ Antimicrobial soap (60% to 95% alcohol or other FDA-approved for surgical hand asepsis).
■ Single-use nail cleaner.
■ Deep sink with foot or knee controls.
■ Shoe covers, cap, and face mask.
■ Sterile gloves.
■ Surgical pack containing sterile towel.

Key Points
■ Don surgical shoe covers, cap, and face mask before the scrub.
■ Remove rings, watches, and bracelets.
■ Using warm water, perform a prewash, using soap and water.
■ Using a pick, clean under your nails, under running water.
■ Keep your hands above your elbows and away from the body.
■ Wet your hands and forearms from fingertips to elbows.
■ Dispense a generous amount of antimicrobial soap.
■ Use a twisting motion for the fingertips and nails. Then vigorously rub the hands together. Scrub all surfaces of nails, fingers, hands, and forearms for the length of time specified by the agency (usually 3 minutes).

The Order of the Scrub Is Generally as Follows:
■ Nondominant hand and fingers, lower ⅓ of nondominant forearm, rinse.
■ Dominant hand and fingers, lower ⅓ of dominant arm, rinse.
■ Repeat the scrub and rinse both hands and lower forearms.
■ Scrub remaining ⅔ of nondominant forearm to 2 in. above elbow, and rinse. Then scrub remaining ⅔ of dominant forearm to 2 in. above elbow, and rinse.
■ Repeat scrub and rinse of upper forearms.
■ Repeat all the preceding scrubbing, stopping before the elbow.
■ Grasp a sterile towel and back away from the sterile field.
■ Thoroughly dry your hands, use one end of the towel for the dominant hand/arm, the other end for the nondominant hand/arm.

Documentation

■ No documentation required. The agency may have a checklist to indicate a scrub was done.

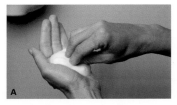

Use a twisting motion for fingertips and nails.

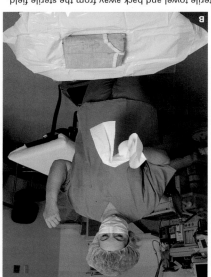

Grasp the sterile towel and back away from the sterile field.

Wilkinson Procedure 20-6. Sterile Gown and Gloves (Closed Method)

✔ For steps to follow in all procedures, refer to the first page of this book, Universal Steps for All Procedures.

Equipment
- Correctly sized sterile gloves.
- Sterile gown.
- **Be Smart!** These should be lying on a sterile field. If not, you must create a sterile field to place them on.

Key Points
- Put on shoe covers, hair covers, and mask before the scrub.
- Perform the surgical scrub and dry your hands well.
- Grasp the gown at the neckline and slide your arms into the sleeves, but not through the cuffs (keep hands inside the sleeves).
- Have a coworker pull the shoulders of your gown up and tie the neck tie for you.
- Don gloves using the closed method by keeping your hands covered at all times, first with the sleeve, then the sterile glove.
- Glove the dominant hand first, then the nondominant hand.
- When gloving, lay the glove on the sleeve-encased forearm thumb side down, with the glove opening pointing toward your fingers.
- Secure the waist tie on your gown by handing it to a coworker and turning to receive it.
- Keep your hands within your field of vision at all times.
- Do not turn your back to a sterile field.

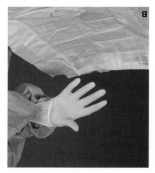

Lay the glove thumb side down, with glove opening pointed toward the fingers.

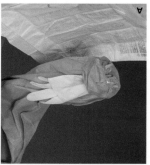

Pull gown sleeve up and move fingers into the glove.

Wilkinson Procedure 20-7. Sterile Gloves (Open Method)

For steps to follow in all procedures, refer to the first page of this book, Universal Steps for All Procedures.

Equipment
- Sterile gloves of the correct size.
- Flat surface to open the package.

Key Points
- Remove all jewelry, including rings and watches.
- Place the glove package on a clean, dry surface.
- Open the inner package so that the cuffs are closest to you.
- Apply the glove of your dominant hand first, touching only the inside of the glove's folded-over cuff with your nondominant hand.
- Apply the second glove by touching only the outer part of the glove with your already-gloved hand; keep your sterile thumb well away from your bare skin.
- Do not touch the gloves to any unsterile items.
- **Be Smart!** Sterile touches sterile; "dirty" touches "dirty."

Documentation
- No special documentation is needed for sterile gloving.
- Record the procedure you perform and the patient's responses.

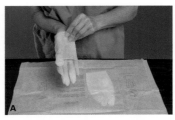

Glove your dominant hand first.

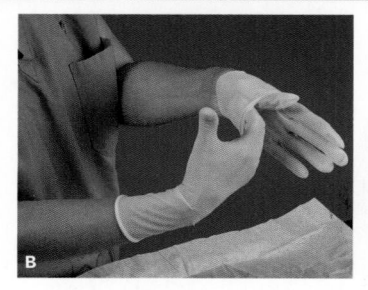

Glove your nondominant hand second.

Wilkinson Procedures 20-8A & B. Setting up a Sterile Field & Adding Supplies to the Sterile Field

✔️ For steps to follow in all procedures, refer to the first page of this book, Universal Steps for All Procedures.

Equipment
- Package of sterile supplies required for the procedure.
- Sterile gloves of the correct size to use in performing the procedure.

Key Points
Setting Up the Sterile Field
- Prepare the sterile field as closely as possible to the time of use.
- Do not cover the sterile field once established.
- Do not turn away from the sterile field.
- Inspect for package integrity, inclusion of sterile indicator, and/or expiration date. Do not use outdated items.
- Clear space; prepare the patient before setting up the sterile field.
- Create the sterile field with a sterile package wrapper or drape.

Adding Supplies to the Sterile Field
- Hold the items several inches above the field.
- Peel back the wrapper.
- Gently drop each item onto the sterile field.

Documentation
- You do not need to document setting up the sterile field.
- Record the procedure you perform, your reassessments of the area being treated, and the patient's tolerance for the procedure.

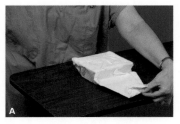

Open the flap away from you first.

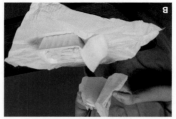

Do not pass your arms over the sterile field as you drop the item.

Wilkinson Procedure 20-8C. Adding Sterile Solutions to a Sterile Field

For steps to follow in all procedures, refer to the first page of this book, Universal Steps for All Procedures.

Equipment
- An established sterile field.
- Sterile bowl or receptacle.
- The correct sterile solution.

Key Points
- Use a sterile bowl or receptacle if the sterile field is fabric or at risk for strike-through.
- Unwrap the sterile bowl and grasp it through the sterile wrapper as you place it near the edge of the sterile field. You may also place the bowl next to, instead of on, the sterile field.
- Confirm that the sterile solution is correct, and that the expiration date has not passed.
- To remove the cap from the solution bottle, lift it directly up. Then discard it.
- Holding the bottle 4 to 6 inches above the bowl, carefully pour the needed amount of the solution into the bowl.
- Discard the remaining solution.
- Before donning sterile gloves to perform the procedure, double-check that all supplies have been added to the field. Do not leave a sterile field unattended. Do not turn your back to the sterile field.

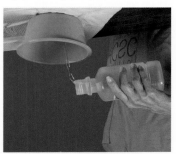

Hold the bottle 4 to 6 in. above the bowl. Pour carefully.

Wilkinson Procedure 21-1. Using a Bed Monitoring Device

✅ For steps to follow in all procedures, refer to the first page of this book, Universal Steps for All Procedures.

Equipment
- Bed or chair exit monitoring device (types: pressure sensitive, posture indicator, motion sensor, and pull-cord alarms).

Assessment
- Identify factors that increase risk for more severe injury in the case of a fall (e.g., anticoagulants, osteoporosis).
- Check the alarm on the monitor to ensure that it is working properly.
- Assess for factors that increase fall risk.
  - *Intrinsic Factors, Examples:*
    - Age > 75.
    - History of falls.
    - Incontinence.
    - Cognitive impairment.
    - Dizziness.
    - Medications.
    - Medical problems (e.g., dementia, arthritis, depression).
  - *Extrinsic (Environmental) Factors, Examples:*
    - Equipment.
    - Wet/uneven floors.
    - Footwear.
    - Poor lighting.
    - Clothing.
    - Lack of grab rails.
    - Furniture/adaptive aids in disrepair (e.g., bed rails).

Post-Procedure Reassessment
- Monitor fall risk per agency policy and as indicated by the patient's physical and mental status.
- If a fall occurs, perform a post-fall assessment to identify possible causes, and monitor more closely for 48 hours.

Key Points

- Select the correct type of alarm for your patient.
- Explain to patient and family that a monitoring device alerts the staff when the patient tries to get out of the chair or bed.
- Apply/place the device; connect the control unit to the sensor pad.
- Connect the control unit to the nurse call system, if possible.
- Explain that the patient will need to call for help when he wants to get up.
- Place the patient on fall risk precautions according to agency policy.
- Assess the sensitivity of the monitoring device, and adjust as needed to ensure that the alarm is activated if the patient tries to get out of the bed or chair.
- Disconnect or turn off the alarm before assisting the patient out of the bed or chair.
- Reactivate the alarm after helping the patient back to the bed or chair.
- **Be Safe!** Bed alarms alone do not prevent falls; they are used to improve the timeliness of staff response. Patients who are at risk for falls require increased observation and surveillance.

Documentation

- Document on the fall risk assessment sheet, restraint flowsheet, and nursing notes according to agency policy.
- Document the initial sensor placement, including type of sensor used and location of placement.
- Follow agency policy for ongoing documentation of the use of a bed exit monitor.
- Usually, the minimum documentation is every 8 hours.

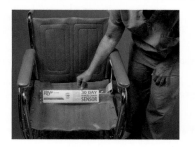

Chair monitor.

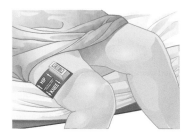

Leg sensor.

Wilkinson Procedure 21-2. Using Restraints

✔️ For steps to follow in all procedures, refer to the first page of this book, Universal Steps for All Procedures.

Equipment
■ Restraint of the appropriate size: belt, vest, wrist, ankle, or mitt.
■ Soft gauze or cotton padding for bony prominences.

Assessment
■ Assess the need for restraints; that is, that the immediate physical safety of the patient, a staff member, or others is threatened.
■ Assess the patient's risk for falls, including mobility status and level of awareness.
■ Determine that all less-restrictive measures have been tried unsuccessfully.
■ Identify the appropriate restraint; one that:
  ■ Is the least restrictive possible.
  ■ Does not interfere with care or exacerbate the patient's medical condition.
  ■ Does not pose a safety risk to the patient.
  ■ Can be changed easily to keep it clean.

Post-Procedure Reassessment
■ Assess the initial restraint placement, circulation, and skin integrity.
■ Check the restraint every 30 minutes (more often for a behavioral restraint). Observe for pallor, cyanosis, and coolness of extremities.
■ Reassess the restraint, circulation, the patient's response to the intervention, and the continuing need for the restraint every 2 hours; remove it as soon as it is no longer needed.

Key Points
■ Follow agency policy, state laws, and professional guidelines.
■ Try alternative interventions first (e.g., bed/chair alarms, patient sitters hired to watch the patient).
■ Use the least restrictive method among the various types of restraints:
  ■ Verbal.
  ■ Chemical (e.g., antipsychotic or sedative medication).
  ■ Seclusion (safe containment to de-escalate).
  ■ Physical (4-point devices, tie-on, Velcro, leather).

- Use restraints only to protect a patient and/or caregiver from injury; not for the convenience of the caregiver or as a punishment.
- Obtain the required consent form.
- Obtain a medical order before restraining, except in an emergency.
- Be Safe! Secure restraints in a way that allows for quick release.
- Be Safe! Tie bed restraints to the bed frame, not to the siderails.
- Be Safe! Ensure that restraints do not impair circulation or tissue integrity.
- Be Safe! Check restraints every 30 minutes.
- Be Smart! A prescriber must reassess and reorder the restraints every 24 hours.
- Release restraints and assess every 2 hours (more often for behavioral restraints).

Documentation

- Document the following on fall risk assessment sheet, restraint flowsheet, and nursing notes per agency policy:
  - All nursing interventions that were done to eliminate the need for the restraint (e.g., moving patient closer to the nurses' station, asking a family member to remain with the patient).
  - Reasons for placing the restraint (e.g., patient behaviors).
  - The initial restraint placement, including location, circulation, and skin integrity.
  - Patient and family teaching.
  - Circulation checks, range of motion, and restraint removal per agency protocol.

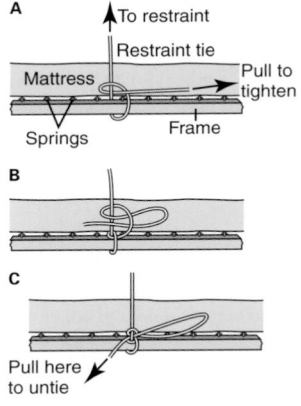

A quick-release knot.

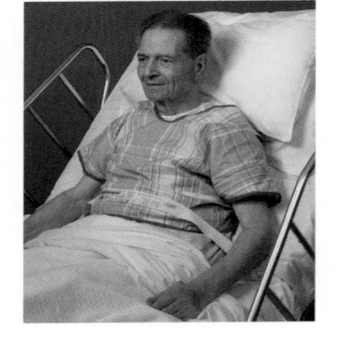

A vest restraint.

Wilkinson Procedure 22-1. Bathing: Providing a Complete Bed Bath

✓ For steps to follow in all procedures, refer to the first page of this book, Universal Steps for All Procedures.

Equipment
- Water basin.
- Bath blanket.
- 2 bath towels.
- Washcloths.
- Soap or liquid rinse-free soap.
- Orangewood stick.
- Deodorant, lotion, and/or powder as needed.
- Clean gown (with shoulder snaps if the patient has an IV line) and bed linen.
- Procedure gloves.
- Bedpan or urinal.
- Laundry bag.
- Be Smart! You may need special soaps and lotions for older adults or patients with skin conditions, or skin breakdown; and additional washcloths and towels for patients with incontinence or drainage.

Assessment
- Assess:
  - Mobility.
  - Activity tolerance.
  - Type of bath needed.
  - Ability to perform bathing self-care.
  - Personal and cultural issues regarding the bath.
  - Specific patient needs and preferences (e.g., special soaps or lotions).
- Check for positioning or activity restrictions.
- Determine how many people you need to safely bathe and reposition the patient.

■ **Be Smart!** Save time. While bathing the patient, assess level of consciousness, short- and long-term memory, ability to follow instructions, ROM, skin condition, activity tolerance, and self-care ability.

Key Points

■ Provide privacy, and offer patient a bedpan before beginning.
■ Use warm, not hot, water (105°F, or 41°C).
■ Protect bed linen with towels unless you will be changing them.
■ Wear procedure gloves if exposure to body fluids (e.g., draining wounds) is likely or if you have breaks in your skin.
■ Prevent chilling or tiring the patient (e.g., cover with bath blanket, expose only the body part you are washing).
■ **Be Safe!** Lower the siderail on the side where you are working; raise it when moving to the other side of the bed.
■ **Be Safe!** Do not disconnect an IV to remove the patient's gown. Remove the gown first from the arm without the IV.
■ Follow the principles, "head to toe" and "clean to dirty" (bathe face, neck, arms and chest, abdomen, legs, feet, back, buttocks, perineum).
■ Change the water and don procedure gloves before cleansing the perineum; change the water whenever it becomes dirty or cool.
■ For extremities, wash and dry from distal to proximal.
■ Pat the skin dry; do not rub.
■ Perform hand hygiene when moving from a contaminated body part to bathe a clean body part.

Documentation

■ You will usually document hygiene care on checklists and flowsheets.
■ For nursing notes, chart:
  ■ The type of bath given.
  ■ Extent to which patient was able to help.
  ■ Tolerance of the procedure.
  ■ Mobility.
  ■ Any abnormal findings.

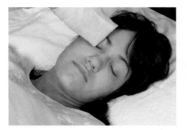

Wipe outward from the inner canthus.

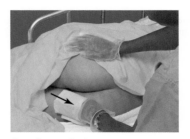

Wash rectal area from front to back.

Wilkinson Procedure 22-4. Providing Perineal Care

✓ For steps to follow in all procedures, refer to the first page of this book, Universal Steps for All Procedures.

Equipment
- Procedure gloves.
- Basin or perineal wash bottle.
- Waterproof pad.
- Bedpan or portable sitz tub (optional).
- Towel.
- Wash cloth.
- Toilet tissue.
- Cleansing solution or soap.
- Perineal ointment if needed.

Assessment
- Assess:
  - Mobility.
  - Activity tolerance.
  - Ability to assist with perineal care.
- Check for positioning or activity restrictions.
- Identify specific needs regarding perineal care (e.g., cultural preferences, presence of a urinary drainage catheter, perineal surgery, or lesions).
- **Be Smart!** If there are lesions or skin breakdown, you may need to use special soaps and/or lotions.
- Incontinence or drainage requires assessment and follow-up to prevent Impaired Skin Integrity.

Key Points
- Provide privacy; keep the patient covered as much as possible.
  - **For females:** Fold a bath blanket into the shape of a diamond. Wrap the side points of the diamond around the patient's legs.
  - **For males:** Place a bath blanket over the chest, then fold bed linens down to expose the groin.
- Place a waterproof pad under the patient to protect the bed linen.
- Use warm water (105°F, or 41°C).
- Follow the principle of "clean to dirty" (front to back for women).

Documentation

- You will usually chart perineal care on a flowsheet.
- For a narrative note, also chart patient responses to the procedure, the condition of the perineal area, and the patient's comfort status.

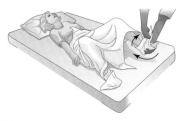

Drape for privacy.

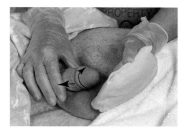

Wash the head of the penis first.

Wilkinson Procedure 22-5. Providing Foot Care

✔ For steps to follow in all procedures, refer to the first page of this book, Universal Steps for All Procedures.

Equipment

■ Procedure gloves (if there are open lesions).
■ Pillow (if procedure is done with the patient in bed).
■ Basin for water.
■ Liquid no-rinse soap.
■ Bath towel.
■ Waterproof pad.
■ Washcloth.
■ Orangewood stick.
■ Toenail clippers.
■ Nail file.
■ Lotion or prescribed ointment or cream.

Assessment

■ Assess:
  ■ Bilateral dorsalis pedis pulses.
  ■ Skin color and warmth.
  ■ All areas of the feet for skin integrity, edema, condition of toenails, abnormalities.
■ Be Smart! Compare right and left feet.
■ Be Smart! Check carefully between the toes.
■ Assess the patient's usual footwear; self-care ability for foot care (including vision and mobility); and knowledge about foot care, including usual foot care practices. Evaluate the need for a referral.
■ Be Smart! Verify that institutional policy allows a nurse to trim toenails. Obtain a prescription, if necessary.

Post-Procedure Reassessment

■ Observe that feet are clean, and smooth; nails are trimmed and smooth; skin is pink, warm, and intact.
■ Identify and provide interventions for foot problems.
■ Ask the patient to demonstrate or describe correct foot care.

Key Points

■ Inspect the feet thoroughly for skin integrity, circulation, and edema.
■ Clean the feet with mild soap; clean the toenails; rinse; and dry well.

- Trim the nails straight across, unless contraindicated or against agency policy
- File the nails with an emery board.
- Lightly apply lotion, except between the toes.
- Ensure that footwear and bedding are not irritating to the feet.

Documentation

- In most agencies, you will not document routine foot care (except, perhaps, on a checklist) unless there are problems.
- If you do document, chart assessment findings and that foot care was given.

Wilkinson Procedure 22-7. Providing Denture Care

☑ For steps to follow in all procedures, refer to the first page of this book, Universal Steps for All Procedures.

Equipment
- Toothbrush or sponge toothettes.
- Denture cleaning paste.
- Emesis basin.
- Towel.
- Glass of water.
- Mouthwash and/or lip moisturizer, if desired.
- Procedure gloves.
- Mask and goggles if splashing may occur.
- Tonsil-tip suction connected to suction source (if aspiration is a concern).
- Denture cup.

Assessment
- Assess:
  - Patient's ability to assist with oral care.
  - General oral health (e.g., presence of the gag reflex and condition of teeth, gums, and mucous membranes).
  - Swallowing ability.
  - Whether the patient has dentures, bridgework, or partial plates.
- Assess patient's usual oral care, including cultural practices.
- Be Smart! If the patient has dentures, examine the mouth with and without the dentures.

Post-Procedure Reassessment
- Check to see that dentures are comfortable and fit properly.
- Inspect the gums and mucous membranes to verify that they are free of food particles.
- Inspect for abnormalities, such as bleeding, that may have been stimulated by mouth care.
- Assess the patient's tolerance of and satisfaction with the care.

Key Points
- If the patient is at risk for choking, suction secretions as needed.
- Remove (and replace) the top denture before the lower denture.

- Tilt dentures slightly when removing and replacing.
- **Be Safe!** Handle dentures carefully, and place the towel in the sink to avoid breaking the dentures if you drop them.
- Use cool water and a stiff-bristled brush; brush all surfaces and rinse thoroughly.
- Apply denture adhesive, if the patient uses it.
- If dentures are dry, moisten them before reinserting.
- Offer mouthwash.

Documentation

- Document that oral care was given, the patient's response, any abnormal findings, and nursing interventions.
- Oral care is usually charted on a flowsheet.

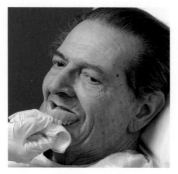

Grasp the top denture with a gauze pad.

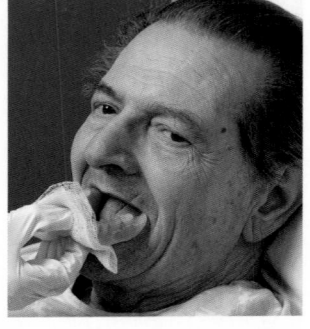

Use thumbs to push up on bottom denture at gumline. Tilt to remove.

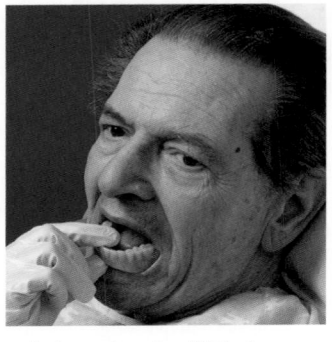

Moisten the denture before reinserting if it is dry.

Wilkinson Procedure 22-8. Providing Oral Care for an Unconscious Patient

For steps to follow in all procedures, refer to the first page of this book, Universal Steps for All Procedures.

Equipment
- Toothbrush with soft bristles or sponge oral swabs.
- Toothpaste.
- Denture cup, if patient has dentures.
- 4 in. × 4 in. gauze pad to remove dentures if present.
- Tonsil-tip suction connected to suction source.
- Tongue blade (padded) or bite-block.
- Towel.
- Waterproof linen protector.
- Emesis basin.
- Water-soluble lip moisturizer.
- Procedure gloves and goggles.

Assessment
- Assess the patient's general oral health, including the condition of the teeth.
- Observe oral mucosa and gums for hydration, inflammation, bleeding, or infection.
- Determine whether the patient has dentures or partial plates. Assess the fit of dentures and the condition of the gums under the dentures.
- Assess the patient's gag reflex.

Post-Procedure Reassessment
- Inspect the teeth, gums, and mucous membranes for cleanliness.
- Observe the patient's overall responses to the procedure (e.g., gagging, coughing, VS, skin color).

Key Points
- Lower the head of the bed unless contraindicated.
- Position the patient side-lying with head turned to the side.
- Place a waterproof pad and towel under the patient's cheek and chin.

- Use a padded tongue blade or bite-block as needed to keep the mouth open.
- Place an emesis basin under the patient's cheek.
- Be Safe! For an unconscious patient, remove partial plates to prevent aspiration.
- Suction secretions as needed.

Documentation

- Document that oral care was given, any abnormal findings, and nursing interventions.
- Typically, oral care is documented on a checklist or flowsheet.

Wilkinson Procedure 22-9B. Shampooing the Hair Using Rinse-Free Shampoo

For steps to follow in all procedures, refer to the first page of this book, Universal Steps for All Procedures.

Equipment
- Rinse-free shampoo (no water is needed).
- Conditioner (optional).
- Bath towel.
- Brush or hair pick.
- Comb.
- Procedure gloves (if scalp lesion or infestation present).

Assessment
- Assess for:
  - Contraindications to a soap-and-water shampoo (e.g., limited head or neck movement, scalp sutures).
  - Ability to assist with the procedure.
  - Condition of the hair and scalp (e.g., dryness or irritation).
- Ask the patient how she normally cares for her hair.
- Be Smart! Assess the need for special hair care products (e.g., dandruff or lice require medicated shampoos; dry hair requires a conditioner).

Post-Procedure Reassessment
- Observe for patient discomfort or fatigue during the procedure.
- Afterward, observe that the hair is clean, dry, and free of tangles.
- Ask the patient how the hair and scalp feel.

Key Points
- Obtain rinse-free shampoo and any other hair care products needed.
- Elevate the head of the bed.
- Place a protective pad or towel under the patient's shoulders.
- Don procedure gloves, and use fingers or a comb to remove tangles.
- Apply enough rinse-free shampoo to thoroughly wet the hair. Work it through the hair, from the scalp down to the ends.
- Towel-dry the hair.

Documentation

■ Chart that hair was shampooed; the method used; the condition of the hair and scalp; and the patient's responses to the procedure.

Wilkinson Procedure 22-14. Making an Occupied Bed

For steps to follow in all procedures, refer to the first page of this book, Universal Steps for All Procedures.

Equipment
- Bottom and top sheets, drawsheet, pillowcase for each of the pillows.
- Bath blanket.
- Linen bag or hamper.
- Procedure gloves (if exposure to body fluids is possible).
- Moisture-proof gown (if heavy soiling of linens with body fluids is possible).

Assessment
- Assess:
  - Ability to move.
  - Need for patient-handling devices.
  - Drainage or incontinence.

Post-Procedure Reassessment
- Assess how well the patient tolerated the procedure (e.g., discomfort, shortness of breath, etc.)
- Ask the patient whether he feels comfortable.

Key Points
- Be Safe! Maintain patient safety during the procedure. Always raise the siderail before moving to the other side of the bed.
- Elevate the bed to working height, position patient laterally near the far siderail, and roll soiled linen under him.
- Place clean linens on the side nearest you, and then tuck under the soiled linen.
- Roll the patient over the "hump," and position him on his other side, near you. Raise the near siderail.
- Move to other side of bed; lower the siderail; pull soiled and clean linen through; and complete the linen change.
- Be Smart! Don't forget to miter corners and make a toe pleat.
- Remove the bath blanket without exposing the patient.
- Be Safe! Place the bed in a low position, raise the siderails, and fasten the call light to the pillow.

Documentation

■ Linen changes are generally recorded on a checklist.
■ A nursing note is needed only if something abnormal occurred.

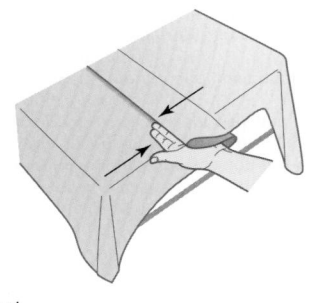

Making a toe pleat.

Wilkinson Procedure 29-1. Performing Otic Irrigation

✅ For steps to follow in all procedures, refer to the first page of this book, Universal Steps for All Procedures.

Equipment
- An ear irrigation system, such as the Welch Allyn ear wash system or an electronic jet ear irrigator.
- Asepto syringe, or rubber bulb syringe (if an ear irrigation system is not available).
- Irrigating solution (usually water, but may be an antiseptic solution), warmed to 98.6°F (37°C).
- Bath towel and moisture-resistant towel.
- A headlight if one is available.
- Emesis basin.
- Otoscope.
- Cotton balls.
- Procedure gloves.
- Be Safe! Do not use a metal syringe, as it is considered dangerous.
- Be Smart! An ear irrigation system is preferred over an Asepto or bulb syringe because of the better ability to control pressure and remove cerumen.

Assessment
- Assess for pain and hearing loss.
- Determine whether there are contraindications for ear irrigation (e.g., recent middle ear infection, cleft palate).
- Assess the external ear for drainage, cerumen.
- Assess the external ear canal for redness, swelling, or foreign objects; visualize the tympanic membrane.
- Be Safe! Do not irrigate if drainage is present or you cannot visualize the tympanic membrane.
- Be Smart! If a foreign object is present, attempt to remove it before irrigation.

Post-Procedure Reassessment
- Observe the quantity and quality of ear cerumen you removed, and the appearance of the ear canal.

- Assess for complaints of pain or dizziness, and for improvement in hearing acuity.
- Observe for drainage on the cotton ball.

Key Points

- Warm the irrigating solution to body temperature.
- Assist the patient into a sitting or lying position, with the head tilted slightly toward the affected ear.
  - **Adults:** Straighten the ear canal by pulling up and back on the pinna.
  - **Young children:** Pull down and back to straighten the canal.
- Instruct the patient to notify you if he experiences any pain or dizziness during the irrigation.
- Place the tip of the nozzle (or syringe) into the entrance of the ear canal, and direct the stream of irrigating solution slowly and gently along the top of the ear canal toward the back of the client's head.
- Continue irrigating until the canal is clean.
- Perform an otoscopic examination.
- Place a cotton ball loosely in the outer ear.

Documentation

- Document:
  - The irrigation solution used.
  - The quantity, character, and odor of cerumen or drainage.
  - The condition of the ear canal and tympanic membrane after the irrigation.

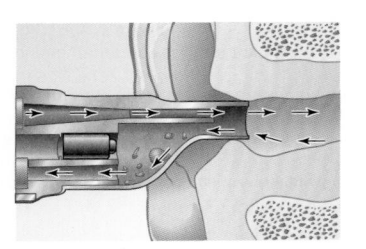

Place the tip of the nozzle about 1 cm (½ in.) above the entrance to the ear canal.

Medication Guidelines: Steps to Follow for All Medications

✔️ For steps to follow in all procedures, refer to the first page of this pocket guide, Universal Steps for All Procedures. When preparing or administering medication, use the following guidelines.

Equipment
- Medication administration record (MAR).
- Medication drawer or portable cart with keys to the medication drawer, as needed.
- Procedure gloves, as needed.
- Other supplies and equipment needed for the specific procedure (e.g., water, alcohol wipes).

Assessment
- Assess for factors that interfere with drug absorption (e.g., diarrhea, inadequate circulation, foods, other drugs).
- Assess for factors that affect metabolism of the drug (e.g., impaired liver function, edema, inflammation, or age-related changes).
- Before the first administration, assess the patient's knowledge about the medications being given.
- Verify the prescribed dosage is appropriate for the patient's age and weight.
- Be Smart! Assess your knowledge of the medication (e.g., drug action, recommended dosage, time of onset and peak action, common side effects, and so on).
- Be Smart! Assess for situations in which administering the medication would not be reasonable (e.g., oral medications prescribed for a patient who is vomiting, who is sedated, or who has difficulty swallowing).
- Be Safe! Before giving the medication, assess VS and check lab studies to determine whether the drug can be safely administered.
- Be Safe! Check for history of allergies to medication or with food.

Post-Procedure Reassessment
- Evaluate the therapeutic effects of the medication.
- Be Safe! Be alert for side effects, allergic reactions, or other adverse reactions. If present, notify the primary care provider.

Key Points

- Observe the "three checks" and the "rights of medication": right patient, drug, dose, time, route, and documentation.
- The prescription should include the patient's name, identifier, medication name, dose, route, time, and allergies.
- Follow agency policies for medication administration, including the time frame for administration.
- Access the patient's medication drawer, unlock the medication cart, or log onto the medication dispensing computer.
- If administering a narcotic or barbiturate, obtain the narcotic cabinet key and sign out the medication, including the patient's name, drug, dose, and other information per agency policy. Note the drug count when removing a narcotic.
- Calculate medication dosage. Double-check it. If you are unable to measure the dose exactly, contact the pharmacist.
- Check the expiration date.
- Lock the medication cart.
- Take the medication and MAR or hand-held portable device with the electronic health record into the patient's room.
- Identify the patient using two forms of identification, according to agency policy.
- Explain to the patient that you are there to administer the medication and teach him about the medication.
- Administer the medication.

Documentation

- Scheduled medications are documented on the MAR.
- Document the name of the medication, time, dose, and route given, and assessments; therapeutic and adverse drug effects, nursing interventions, and teaching.
- Record PRN medications in the nursing notes; include reason given and response.
- For parenteral medications, note the site of injection.
- **Be Smart!** When a drug is not administered, document that on the MAR along with the reason. Inform the prescriber.
- **Be Safe!** Do not document before giving the drug. Do not document for anyone else or ask them to document for you.

Wilkinson Procedure 23-1. Administering Oral Medication

For steps to follow in all procedures, refer to the first page of this pocket guide, Universal Steps for All Procedures. When administering medication, also follow the guidelines in Medication Guidelines: Steps to follow for All Medications at the beginning of this section of this pocket guide.

Equipment
- MAR.
- Medication drawer or portable cart with keys to the medication drawer, as needed.
- Procedure gloves, as needed.
- Other supplies and equipment needed for the specific procedure (e.g., water, alcohol wipes).

Assessment
- Assess for factors that interfere with drug absorption (e.g., diarrhea, inadequate circulation, foods, other drugs).
- Assess for factors that affect absorption and/or metabolism of the drug (e.g., impaired liver function, edema, inflammation, or age-related changes).
- Before the first administration, assess the patient's knowledge about the medications being given.
- Be Smart! Assess your knowledge of the medication (e.g., drug action, recommended dosage, time of onset and peak action, common side effects, and so on); and verify the prescribed dosage is appropriate for the patient's age and weight.
- Be Safe! Before giving the medication, assess VS and check lab studies to determine whether the drug can be safely administered.
- Be Smart! Assess for situations in which administering the medication would not be reasonable (e.g., oral medications prescribed for a patient who is vomiting, who is sedated, or who has difficulty swallowing).
- Be Safe! Check for history of allergies.

Post-Procedure Reassessment
- Evaluate the therapeutic effects of the medication. For example, check BP after administering an antihypertensive medication, or check pain level after an analgesic.

■ **Be Safe!** Be alert for side effects, allergic reactions, or other adverse reactions. If present, notify the primary care provider.

Key Points

■ Observe the "three checks" and the "rights of medication": right patient, drug, dose, time, route, and documentation.
  ■ **Tablets and capsules:** Count the correct number aloud.
  ■ **Liquids:** Hold the medication cup at eye level to measure the dose.
■ Assist the patient to a high-Fowler's position, if possible.
■ Administer the medication:
  ■ **Powder:** Mix with liquid, and give it to the patient to drink.
  ■ **Lozenge:** Instruct the patient not to chew or swallow it before it dissolves in her mouth.
  ■ **Tablet or capsule:** Place the tablet in her mouth or hand, or in a medication cup; instruct the patient to swallow with sips of liquid.
  ■ **Sublingual:** Instruct the patient to place the tablet under the tongue and hold it there until it is completely dissolved.
  ■ **Buccal:** Instruct the patient to place the tablet between the cheek and teeth and hold it there until it is completely dissolved.

Documentation

■ Scheduled medications are documented on the MAR.
■ Document:
  ■ Medication, time, dose, and route given, and assessments.
  ■ Therapeutic and adverse drug effects.
  ■ Nursing interventions.
  ■ Teaching.
■ Record PRN medications in the nursing notes; include reason given and response.
■ For parenteral medications, note the site of injection.

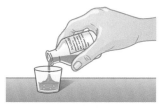

Hold the bottle with the label in your palm.

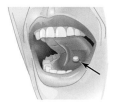

Sublingual—Place and hold the tablet under the tongue until it is completely dissolved.

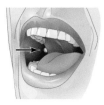

Buccal—Place the tablet between the cheek and teeth or tongue.

Wilkinson Procedure 23-1A. Administering Medication Through an Enteral Tube

✔ For steps to follow in all procedures, refer to the first page of this pocket guide, Universal Steps for All Procedures. When administering medication, also follow the guidelines in Medication Guidelines: Steps to follow for All Medications at the beginning of this section of this pocket guide.

Equipment
- Procedure gloves.
- Water (for diluting and flushing the feeding tube).
- 60-mL catheter-tip syringe.
- Stethoscope (e.g., to check the apical pulse before administering some cardiac medications).

Assessment
- For NG tubes, check tube placement by aspirating stomach contents or measuring the pH of the aspirate, if possible.
- Other, less accurate, methods are injecting air into the feeding tube and auscultating, or asking the patient to speak.
- Be Safe! Never rely on only one bedside method for checking tube placement; use a combination of methods.

Post-Procedure Reassessment
- Evaluate the therapeutic effects of the medication.
- Be Safe! Be alert for adverse reactions, side effects, or allergic reactions. If present, notify the appropriate care provider.

Key Points
- If the patient is receiving a continuous tube feeding, disconnect it before giving the medications. Leave the tube clamped for a few minutes after administering the medication, according to agency protocol.
- Prepare the medication.
- Give the liquid form of medication, if possible. If the solution is hypertonic, dilute with 10 to 30 mL of sterile water before instilling through a feeding tube.
- Be Smart! If pills must be given, verify that the medication can be crushed and given through an enteral tube.
  - Crush the tablet and mix it with about 20 mL of water.

- If you are giving several medications, mix and administer each one separately and flush afterward.
- Don nonsterile procedure gloves.
- Place patient in a sitting (high-Fowler's) position, if possible.
- Check for residual volume.
- Flush the tube. Based on the type of tube, use a piston tip or Luer-Lok syringe. Remove the bulb or plunger; attach the barrel to the tube; and pour in 20 to 30 mL of water.
- Depress the syringe plunger or using the barrel of the syringe as a funnel and pour in the medication. A smaller tube or thicker medication will require use of a 30- to 60-mL syringe.
- Flush the medication through the tube by instilling more water.
- Have the patient maintain a sitting position for at least 30 minutes after you administer the medication.

Documentation
- Document:
  - Medication, time, dose, and route given, assessments.
  - Therapeutic and adverse drug effects, nursing interventions, and teaching.
  - Patency, residual volume, and placement of tube.
  - Any difficulty with administering the medications.
- Record scheduled medications on the MAR and PRN medications in the nursing notes. For PRN medications, include reason given and response.
- When a drug is not administered, document that on the MAR along with the reason, and inform the prescriber.
- Be Smart! Document on the I&O record the amount of liquid medication and the water used for swallowing medication or flushing the tube.
- Some providers prescribe a specific amount of water to flush with each medication or feeding.

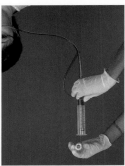

Instilling medication through an enteral tube.

Wilkinson Procedure 23-2. Administering Ophthalmic Medication

✔ For steps to follow in all procedures, refer to the first page of this pocket guide, Universal Steps for All Procedures. When administering medication, also follow the guidelines in Medication Guidelines: Steps to follow for All Medications at the beginning of this section of this pocket guide.

Equipment
- Eye drops or ointment.
- Tissue.

Assessment
- Assess the eyes for redness, drainage, or other signs of irritation or pain.
- Determine the patient's ability to cooperate with the procedure.
- Assess whether the eyes need to be cleansed before administration of the medication.
- Be Safe! Check the prescription for where to instill medication. (Note: We do not advise using these abbreviations—they have been disallowed by The Joint Commission—but you may still see them written in prescriptions: OD = right eye; OS = left eye; OU = both eyes.)

Key Points
- Use a high-Fowler's position, with the head slightly tilted back.
- Work from the inner to outer canthus when cleansing or instilling medication.
- Apply the medication into the conjunctival sac.
- Be Safe! Do not apply the medication to the cornea.
- Be Smart! Do not let the dropper or tube touch the eye.
- For eye drops, press gently against the same side of the nose for 1 to 2 minutes to close the lacrimal ducts.
- For eye ointment, ask the patient to gently close the eyes for 2 to 3 minutes.

Documentation
- Document:
  - Medication, time, dose, and route given.
  - Assessment.
  - Therapeutic and adverse drug effects.

   ■ Nursing interventions, and teaching.
   ■ Assessment data before, during, and after instillation.
■ **Be Safe!** Record scheduled medications on the MAR and PRN medications in the nursing notes. For PRN medications, include reason given and response.
■ **Be Smart!** When a drug is not administered, document that on the MAR along with the reason, and inform the prescriber.
■ **Be Safe!** Do not document before giving the drug. Do not document for anyone else or ask them to document for you.

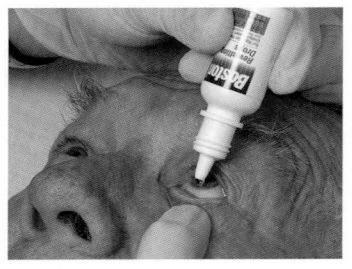

Instilling ophthalmic drops into the eye.

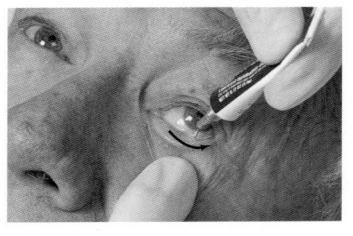

Instilling ophthalmic ointment into the eye.

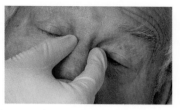

Press lacrimal ducts to reduce systemic absorption.

Wilkinson Procedure 23-3. Administering Otic Medication

For steps to follow in all procedures, refer to the first page of this pocket guide, Universal Steps for All Procedures. When administering medication, also follow the guidelines in Medication Guidelines: Steps to follow for All Medications at the beginning of this section of this pocket guide.

Equipment
- Ear drops.
- Dropper with flexible rubber tip.
- Cotton-tipped applicators.
- Cotton ball.

Assessment
- Assess the external ear and canal for erythema, drainage, and cerumen.
- Assess for ear pain or hearing impairment.

Post-Procedure Reassessment
- Assess for discomfort or pain during the procedure and for relief afterward.
- Evaluate for wax build-up, redness, swelling, or drainage.

Key Points
- Warm the solution to be instilled.
  - **Be Safe!** Do not exceed body temperature.
- Assist the patient to a side-lying position, with the affected ear facing up.
- Straighten the ear canal. For an adult, pull the pinna up and back; for a child 3 years or younger, down and back.
- Instill the ordered number of drops into the ear canal.
  - **Be Safe!** Do not force the solution into the ear or occlude the ear canal with the dropper.
- Instruct the patient to remain on his side for 5 to 10 minutes.

Documentation
- Record:
  - Medication, time, dose, and route given, and signature.
  - Amount, color, character, and odor of any drainage.

- Swelling or redness in the ear canal.
- Pain or discomfort and hearing loss.
- Therapeutic and adverse drug effects, nursing interventions, and teaching.
■ Document scheduled medications on the MAR, and PRN medications in the nursing notes (along with reason given and response).
■ Chart assessments before, during, and after instillation.

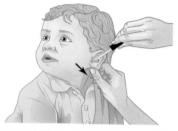

For infants and young children, pull pinna down and back.

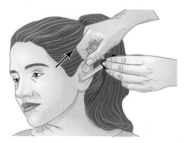

For instilling drops into an adult's ear, pull pinna up and back.

Wilkinson Procedure 23-4. Administering Nasal Medication

☑ For steps to follow in all procedures, refer to the first page of this pocket guide, Universal Steps for All Procedures. When administering medication, also follow the guidelines in Medication Guidelines: Steps to follow for All Medications at the beginning of this section of this pocket guide.

Equipment
- Medication drops, spray, or aerosol.
- Tissues.

Assessment
- Check for nasal obstruction and congestion.
- Assess nasal discharge for color, consistency, and odor. Note the color of nasal drainage.
- Assess nasal mucous membranes for redness, color, moisture, excoriation, or trauma.

Post-Procedure Reassessment
- Assess for symptom relief 15 to 20 minutes after administration.

Key Points
- Determine head position: Consider the indication for the medication and the patient's ability to assume the position.
- Explain to the patient that the medication may cause some burning, tingling, or unusual taste.
- Position the patient with the head down and forward (for sprays) or supine with the head back (for drops).
- Place the tip of the sprayer into the nostril, pointing the tip toward the outside of the nose (toward the outside corner of the right eye).
  - **Be Safe!** Never point the tip toward the middle of the nose (the septum) or straight up (toward the sinus).
- Have the patient blow his nose, occlude one nostril, and exhale.
- Squirt the spray into the nose while the patient inhales through his other nostril. Repeat for the other nostril.

Documentation

- Record:
  - Premedication assessment.
  - Type and amount of solution administered, route.
  - Any patient discomfort during the procedure.
  - Patient's report of response to the medication, (e.g., nasal discharge, obstruction, bleeding, or other complication).

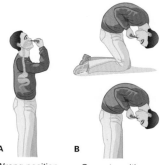

A
Wrong position

B
Correct positions

Instilling nose spray.

Wilkinson Procedure 23-5. Administering Vaginal Medication

✔️ For steps to follow in all procedures, refer to the first page of this pocket guide, Universal Steps for All Procedures. When administering medication, also follow the guidelines in Medication Guidelines: Steps to follow for All Medications at the beginning of this section of this pocket guide.

Equipment
- Medication (foam, jelly, cream, suppository, douche, or irrigating solution).
- Applicator (if indicated).
- Washcloth and warm water for perineal care as needed.
- Water-soluble lubricant.
- Toilet tissue.
- Perineal pad.
- Bath blanket.
- *For irrigation:*
  - Waterproof pad.
  - Bedpan.
  - Vaginal irrigation set (may be disposable; consists of a solution container, nozzle, tubing, and clamp).
  - IV pole.

Assessment
- Assess for:
  - Vaginal burning.
  - Pruritis.
  - Pain.

Post-Procedure Reassessment
- Assess for:
  - Purulent vaginal discharge.
  - Vaginal burning.
  - Pruritis.
  - Pain.

Key Points
For Vaginal Suppository
- Position the patient in a dorsal recumbent or Sims' position.
- Inspect and cleanse the vaginal area.
- Apply a water-soluble lubricant to the rounded end of the suppository and to the gloved index finger on your dominant hand.
- Separate the labia with your nondominant hand.
- Insert the suppository or applicator into the vagina along the posterior vaginal wall about 8 cm (3 in.).
- Instruct the patient to maintain the position for 5 to 15 minutes.

Applicator Insertion of Cream, Foam, or Jelly
- Position the patient in a dorsal recumbent or Sims' position.
- Inspect and cleanse the vaginal area.
- Separate the labia with your nondominant hand.
- Insert the applicator approximately 8 cm (3 in.) into the vagina along the posterior vaginal wall.
- Depress the plunger on the applicator. Dispose of the applicator. If it is reusable, place it on a paper towel and wash it later with soap and water.
- Instruct the patient to remain in a supine position for 5 to 15 minutes.

For Irrigation (Douche)
- Inspect and cleanse the vaginal area.
- Warm the irrigation solution to approximately 105°F (40.6°C).
- Hang the irrigation solution approximately 30 to 60 cm (1 to 2 ft) above the level of the patient's vagina.
- Position the patient in a dorsal recumbent position on a waterproof pad and bedpan.
- Insert the nozzle approximately 7 to 8 cm (3 in.) into the vagina, and start the flow of irrigation solution.

Documentation
- Document:
  - Medication, time, dose, and route given.
  - Therapeutic and adverse drug effects, nursing interventions, and teaching.
  - Condition of vaginal tissue and perineal area, if abnormalities are present.

- Any complaints of discomfort outside of the expected range.
- Length of time the suppository was retained.
- For vaginal irrigations, chart:
  - Assessment.
  - Type and amount of solution administered.
  - Patient discomfort during the procedure.
  - Patient's report of decreased vaginal pain, itching, and/or burning following the procedure.

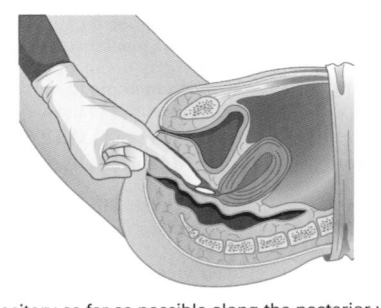

Insert the suppository as far as possible along the posterior vaginal wall.

Wilkinson Procedure 23-6. Inserting a Rectal Suppository

✔ For steps to follow in all procedures, refer to the first page of this pocket guide, Universal Steps for All Procedures. When administering medication, also follow the guidelines in Medication Guidelines: Steps to follow for All Medications at the beginning of this section of this pocket guide.

Equipment
- Suppository.
- Water-soluble lubricant.
- Toilet tissue.

Assessment
- Assess the rectal area for hemorrhoids or irritation.
- Be Smart! Before inserting the suppository, assess for contraindications, such as rectal surgery, rectal bleeding, or cardiac disease.

Post-Procedure Reassessment
- Assess for pain or burning during insertion of the medication.
- Determine that the patient retained the suppository for the desired length of time (reinsertion may be required).
- Assess for rectal pain, if indicated.

Key Points
- Position the client in Sims' position.
- Lubricate the suppository.
- Insert the suppository past the internal sphincter about ½ to 1 in. in infants and 1 to 3 in. in adults.
- Be Safe! Never force the suppository during insertion.
- Instruct the patient to stay on his side for 5 to 10 minutes and to retain (not expel) the suppository for about 30 minutes.

Documentation
- Document:
  - Medication, time, dose, and route given.
  - Therapeutic and adverse drug effects, nursing interventions, and teaching.
  - Condition of anal tissue if abnormalities are present.
  - Any complaints of discomfort outside of the expected range.
  - Length of time the suppository was retained.

- Record assessment data before, during, and after administering the suppository.
- Record PRN medications in the nursing notes, including reason given and response.

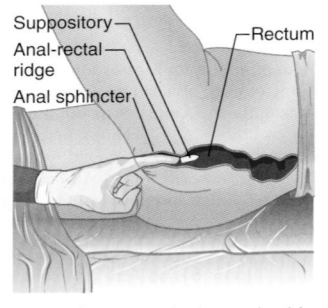

Inserting the rectal suppository past the internal sphincter.

Wilkinson Procedure 23-7D. Applying Transdermal Medication

✓ For steps to follow in all procedures, refer to the first page of this pocket guide, Universal Steps for All Procedures. When administering medication, also follow the guidelines in Medication Guidelines: Steps to follow for All Medications at the beginning of this section of this pocket guide.

Equipment
■ Procedure gloves.
■ Transdermal medication.

Assessment
■ Assess for skin irritation, open lesions, area of hypersensitivity, or other skin abnormality.
■ Determine the presence of contraindications for dermal application.

Post-Procedure Reassessment
■ Assess for rash, excoriation, hives, redness, swelling.
■ Ask the patient if he feels burning, itching, pain, tenderness, or other sensation to skin where medication was applied.

Key Points
■ Be Smart! Wear gloves to avoid absorbing the medication through your own skin and to avoid cross-contamination.
■ Remove the previous patch, folding the medicated side to the inside.
■ Dispose of the old patch carefully in a biohazard receptacle, keeping it away from children and pets.
■ Use soap and water to cleanse the skin of traces of remaining medication. Allow the skin to dry.
■ Remove the new patch from its protective covering, and then remove the clear, protective covering without touching the adhesive or the inside surface that contains the medication.
■ Apply the patch to a clean, dry, hairless (or little hair), intact skin area, pressing it down for about 10 seconds with your palm.
■ Rotate application sites. Common sites are the trunk, lower abdomen, lower back, and buttocks.

- Remove gloves and wash your hands again.
- **Be Safe!** Teach the patient to not use a heating pad over the area.
- **Be Safe!** Do not apply medication to skin with open lesions, irritation, or known hypersensitivity.
- Teach the patient to avoid exposure to ultraviolet light/sunlight after applying medication.
- Use gentle technique when applying topical medication to fragile skin, which is typical in older adults. Take care to not over-apply the medication.

Documentation

- Record scheduled medications in the MAR.
- Record PRN medications in the nursing notes, including the reason given and response.
- Record medication, time, dose, and route given; condition of skin if abnormalities are present, and complaints of discomfort during or after administration.
- Document responses to medication (e.g., symptom relief, side effects); therapeutic and adverse drug effects, nursing interventions, and teaching.
- Document assessment data before, during, and after instillation.

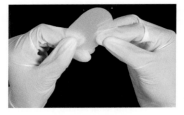

Removing the clear, protective covering from a transdermal patch without touching the adhesive or the inside surface.

Wilkinson Procedure 23-8. Administering Metered-Dose Inhaler Medication

✔️ For steps to follow in all procedures, refer to the first page of this pocket guide, Universal Steps for All Procedures. When administering medication, also follow the guidelines in Medication Guidelines: Steps to follow for All Medications at the beginning of this section of this pocket guide.

Equipment
- MDI.
- Spacer.
- Tissues.

Assessment
- Assess respiratory status before administration of medication to establish a baseline for evaluating the effects of treatment.

Post-Procedure Reassessment
- Be Safe! Assess for change in respiratory status, including VS, and oxygen saturation.

Key Points
- Be Smart! Identify the number of remaining inhalations in the canister. The "float method" is no longer recommended for determining whether an MDI canister is empty.
- Shake the inhaler. Remove the mouthpiece cap of the inhaler and insert the mouthpiece into the spacer while holding the canister upright.
- Remove the cap from the spacer.
- Ask the patient to breathe out slowly and completely.
- If the patient is unable to use the MDI independently, time the use of the device with the patient's respirations.
- Place the spacer mouthpiece into the patient's mouth and ask him to seal his lips around the mouthpiece. Press down on the inhaler canister to discharge one puff of medication into the spacer.
- Ask the patient to slowly inhale through the nose; then hold his breath for as long as possible.
- If a second puff is needed, wait at least 1 minute and repeat.

Documentation

- Chart scheduled medications in the MAR.
- Chart PRN medications in the nursing notes, including reason given and response.
- Record medication, time, dose, and route given; therapeutic and adverse drug effects, nursing interventions, and teaching.
- Document assessment data before, during, and after instillation.

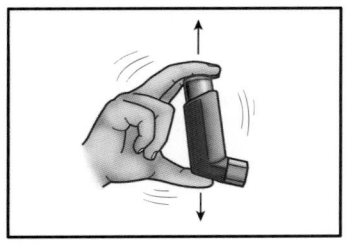

Step 1: Shake the canister.

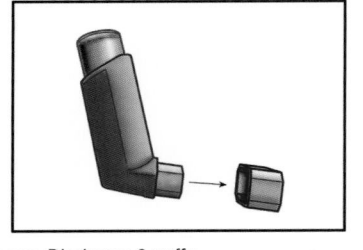

Step 2: Remove cap. Discharge 2 puffs.

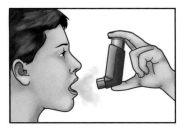

Step 3: Deep breath out.

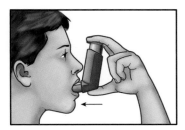

Step 4: Press top. Inhale medication slowly.

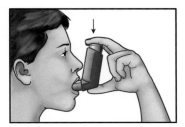

Step 5: Hold breath. Exhale slowly.

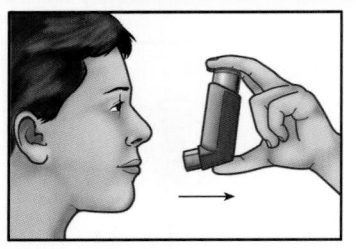

Step 6: Remove inhaler from mouth. Wait 1 minute before next puff.

Wilkinson Procedure 23-9B. Preparing, Drawing Up, and Mixing Medication (One Ampule & One Vial)

For steps to follow in all procedures, refer to the first page of this pocket guide, Universal Steps for All Procedures. When administering medication, also follow the guidelines in Medication Guidelines: Steps to follow for All Medications at the beginning of this section of this pocket guide.

Equipment
- Medication vials, ampules, and/or prefilled syringe.
- Alcohol prep pad (70% alcohol) or CHG-alcohol product.
- Syringe of the appropriate size for medication volume and viscosity.
- VAD, filter needle, or safety needle.
- Gauze pad or ampule snapper.

Assessment
- Check that the ampule and vial are intact, and that the medication is clear, with no discoloration, cloudiness, or particles.

Post-Procedure Reassessment
- Assess for a change in color, cloudiness, particles in the medication mixed.

Key Points
- **Be Smart!** Before beginning, determine the total volume of all medications to be put in the syringe and whether that volume is appropriate for the administration site.
- **Be Safe!** Make sure the medications are compatible.
- Maintain the sterility of the needles and medication.
- **Be Smart!** When drawing up from a single-dose vial and ampule, draw up from the vial first.
- Scrub the stopper of a multidose vial using an alcohol wipe or CHG-alcohol product. Use povidone-iodine only when there is sensitivity to alcohol.
- Draw up the same volume of air as the dose of medication ordered for the vial.
- Inject air into the vial, being careful not to let the needle enter the fluid.
- Then invert the vial and withdraw the dose; expel the air bubbles; and, when the dose is correct, withdraw the needle from the vial.

- **Be Safe!** When opening ampules, protect yourself from injury by using an ampule snapper, folded gauze pad, or still-wrapped alcohol wipe.
- Attach a filter needle or straw to withdraw medication from ampules; change to a needle of the proper length and gauge for administering the medication.
- Flick or tap the top of the ampule to remove medication from the neck of the ampule.
- Open the ampule by wrapping the neck with a folded gauze pad or an unopened alcohol wipe or use an ampule snapper. Snap open away from you.
- Withdraw the second medication very carefully because the medications are mixed as you pull back the plunger; therefore, you must withdraw the exact amount. If there is any excess, you must discard the contents of the syringe and start over. You must avoid contaminating a multidose vial with the second medication.
- Draw 0.2 mL of air into the syringe.
- Confirm the dose is correct by holding the syringe vertically and checking the dose at eye level.
- **Be Smart!** Always recap a sterile needle using a safety capping device or the one-handed scoop method.

Documentation

- Document per MAR, according to agency policy.

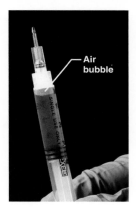

Air
bubble

Incorrect—If the syringe is not vertical, air is trapped.

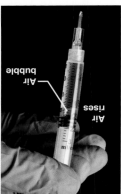

Incorrect—If the tip is down and the syringe is not vertical, air is trapped at the plunger.

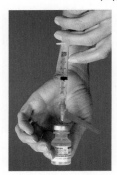

Correct—Syringe is vertical.

Wilkinson Procedure 23-10A. Recapping Needles Using One-Handed Technique (Contaminated Needles)

✅ For steps to follow in all procedures, refer to the first page of this pocket guide, Universal Steps for All Procedures. When administering medication, also follow the guidelines in Medication Guidelines: Steps to follow for All Medications at the beginning of this section of this pocket guide.

Equipment
- Mechanical recapping device, if available.
- Needle cover.
- Safety syringe, if available.
- Other supplies depending on the method used.

Key Points
- Be Safe!
- Recap a contaminated needle only if you cannot avoid it.
- Do not place either of your hands near the needle cap when recapping the needle or engaging the safety mechanism.
- If you are using a safety needle, engage the safety mechanism to cover the needle.
- Place the needle cap in a mechanical recapping device if one is available.
- If recapping devices are not available and you must recap the needle for your own and/or the patient's safety, use the one-handed scoop technique.

Documentation
- No documentation needed for recapping needles.

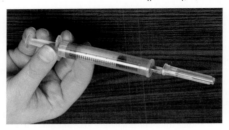

Place needle cover on flat surface.

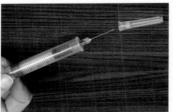

Scoop the cap onto the needle.

Wilkinson Procedure 23-11. Administering Intradermal Medication

✅ For steps to follow in all procedures, refer to the first page of this pocket guide, Universal Steps for All Procedures. When administering medication, also follow the guidelines in Medication Guidelines: Steps to follow for All Medications at the beginning of this section of this pocket guide.

Equipment
- 1-mL syringe (tuberculin) with intradermal needle (25- to 28-gauge, ¼- to ⅝-inch with short bevel).
- Alcohol prep pad or CHG-alcohol product.
- 2 in. × 2 in. gauze pad; pen (ink or felt).

Assessment
- Assess for previous reaction to skin testing and for all types of allergies.
- Assess the skin at intradermal sites for bruising, swelling, tenderness, and other abnormalities.
- Be Safe! Do not give intradermal skin tests if skin abnormalities are present. Also avoid giving them in areas where reading the results may be difficult, such as areas of heavy hair growth.

Post-Procedure Reassessment
- Reassess 5 and 15 minutes after administration for allergic reactions.
- Read the site within 48 to 72 hours of injection, depending on the test.
- Observe that a wheal (about 6 to 8 mm in diameter) forms at the site and that it gradually disappears.
- Observe for minimal bruising that may develop at the site of injection.

Key Points
- Be Safe! Have appropriate antidotes for certain injections readily available before beginning the procedure.
- Be Safe! Know the location of resuscitation equipment in case of a life-threatening adverse reaction.
- Be Safe! Maintain sterile technique and standard precautions.
- Be Smart! Be aware that an intradermal dose is small, usually about 0.01 to 0.1 mL.

- Use a 1-mL syringe and a 25- to 28-gauge, ¼- to ⅝-inch needle.
- Choose a site on the ventral surface of the forearm, upper back, or upper chest.
- Hold the syringe parallel to the skin at a 5° to 15° angle with the bevel up.
- Stretch the skin taut to insert the needle.
- Do not aspirate.
- Inject slowly, and create a wheal or bleb.
- Do not massage or bandage the site.

Documentation

- Document medication, time, dose, and route given, lot numbers (check agency policy), and when the test is to be read.
- Chart therapeutic and adverse drug effects, nursing interventions, and teaching.
- Record scheduled medications on the MAR and PRN medications in the nursing notes.
- For PRN medications, include reason given and response.

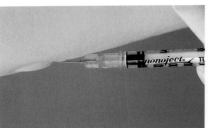

Injecting intradermal medication.

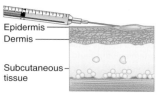

Epidermis

Dermis

Subcutaneous tissue

Inject at a 5° to 15° angle.

Wilkinson Procedure 23-12. Administering Subcutaneous Medication

For steps to follow in all procedures, refer to the first page of this pocket guide, Universal Steps for All Procedures. When administering medication, also follow the guidelines in Medication Guidelines: Steps to follow for All Medications at the beginning of this section of this pocket guide.

Equipment
- Syringe and needle appropriate for volume and site.
- Alcohol prep pad or CHG-alcohol product.
- Gauze pad (optional).

Assessment
- Check the area for previous injection sites.
- Do focused assessments for the specific medication being administered.
- *Insulin*—Be Safe! Check capillary blood sugar level, and determine when the patient will be having the next meal; check for signs of hypoglycemia or hyperglycemia.
- *Heparin*—Check aPTT and for signs of bleeding (e.g., bleeding from gums, IV sites, and so on).

Post-Procedure Reassessment
- Reassess for anticipated response and adverse reaction to the medication.
- Be Smart! *For insulin,* check blood glucose levels and clinical signs that patient's blood sugar level has returned to normal. *For heparin,* observe that patient has no signs of bleeding.

Key Points
- Maintain sterile technique and standard precautions.
- Usually you will use a 1-mL syringe and a 25- to 27-gauge needle that is less than 1 in. long (usually ⅜ to ⅝ in.) For doses of a full mL or more (especially medications other than insulin or heparin), use a 3-mL syringe so you will be better able to aspirate.
- Be Safe! A subcutaneous dose is typically no more than 1 mL.
- Most common injection sites: outer aspect of the upper arms, abdomen, and anterior aspects of the thighs.

- Pinch the skin to inject, as a general rule.
- For an average-weight or thin client, inject at a 45° angle; for an obese client, inject at a 90° angle, as a general rule.
- Aspiration is optional for most subcutaneous medications, but do not aspirate when injecting heparin or insulin.
- Be Safe! Do not massage the site.

Documentation
- Document scheduled medications on the MAR.
- Document PRN medications in the nursing notes, including the reason given and response.
- Chart medication, time, dose, and route given; therapeutic and adverse drug effects, nursing interventions, and teaching.
- Some agencies have a specific code for documenting subcutaneous injections, which allows exact site documentation on an outline of the body.
- In nursing notes, document any related patient assessment findings, such as capillary blood sugar, signs of hypoglycemia or hyperglycemia, bruising, and so on.

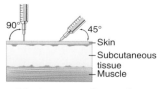

Subcutaneous tissue injection using 45° and 90° angles.

Wilkinson Procedure 23-13. Locating Intramuscular Injection Sites

✔️ For steps to follow in all procedures, refer to the first page of this pocket guide, Universal Steps for All Procedures. When administering medication, also follow the guidelines in Medication Guidelines: Steps to follow for All Medications at the beginning of this section of this pocket guide.

Assessment
■ Be Safe! Always palpate the landmarks and the muscle mass to ensure correct placement of the needle.

Key Points
Ventrogluteal Site
■ Ask the patient to assume a side-lying position with the legs straight, if possible. Alternatively, use a supine position.
■ On adults, the site is a triangle formed between your fingers when you place your palm on the head of the trochanter, index finger on the anterior superior iliac spine, and middle finger pointing toward the iliac crest.

Deltoid Site
■ Be Safe! Completely expose the patient's upper arm.
■ Remove the garment; do not roll up the sleeve. Incomplete exposure of site and landmarks creates a risk of injecting into other than muscle tissue.
■ Locate the lower edge of the acromion process (knobby part of shoulder), and go two to three fingerbreadths down (3 to 5 cm).
■ Draw an imaginary line from the anterior axillary crease to the posterior axillary cease. The deltoid site is the resulting inverted triangle.
■ An alternative approach is to place four fingerbreadths across the deltoid muscle, with your top finger on the acromion process. The injection goes three fingerbreadths below the process in the midline of the upper arm.

Vastus Lateralis Site
■ Be Smart! Position the patient lying supine or sitting. The patient may perceive the injection as less painful if supine because he cannot see the needle enter his leg. For some people this provokes anxiety and intensifies pain.

- Locate the greater trochanter and the lateral femoral condyle.
- Midlateral thigh: On adults, one handbreadth below the head of the trochanter and one handbreadth above the knee. The site is the middle third of this area, slightly lateral to the midline of the anterior thigh.
- **Be Safe!** The vastus lateralis site is safe for patients of all ages and is the recommended site for children younger than 7 months.

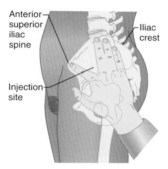

Anterior superior iliac spine

Iliac crest

Injection site

Locating the ventrogluteal site.

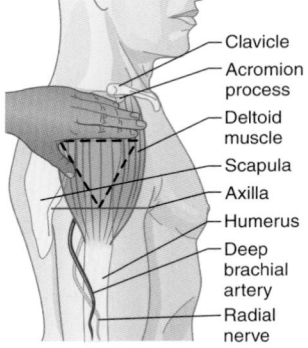

Locating the deltoid site.

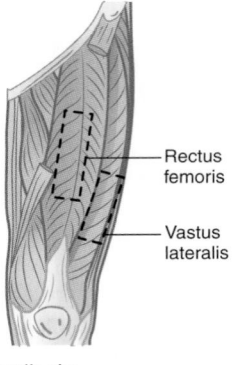

Locating the vastus lateralis site.

Wilkinson Procedure 23-14B. Intramuscular Injection: Z-Track Method

✔️ For steps to follow in all procedures, refer to the first page of this pocket guide, Universal Steps for All Procedures. When administering medication, also follow the guidelines in Medication Guidelines: Steps to follow for All Medications at the beginning of this section of this pocket guide.

Equipment
- Syringe and needle appropriate for volume and site.
- Alcohol prep pad or CHG-alcohol product.
- Gauze pad or adhesive bandage.
- Medication.
- Procedure gloves.
- Biohazard (sharps) container.
- Small piece of gauze or cotton ball.
- Small adhesive bandage.

Assessment
- Identify the site of the previous injection.
- Assess the site for adequate muscle mass, bruises, edema, tenderness, redness, or other abnormalities.
- Assess for factors that affect absorption of the medication (e.g., decreased IM blood flow, as found in shock).

Post-Procedure Reassessment
- Observe for bruising or oozing at the site of injection.
- Observe for local reactions at site (e.g., pain, swelling, redness).

Key Points
- Maintain sterile technique and standard precautions.
- Use a 1- to 5-mL syringe and a 21- to 25-gauge, 1- to 3-in. needle (longer needle if the patient is obese).
- The usual volume per injection is no more than 3 mL.
- Select an appropriate injection site; identify the site using anatomical landmarks.
- Be Smart! The ventrogluteal site is preferred. The deltoid site is acceptable for smaller doses and adult vaccines.

- **Be Smart!** When giving more than one injection, rotate sites.
- Position the patient so that the injection site is well exposed and the patient is able to relax the appropriate muscles. Ensure good lighting.
- Cleanse the site with an antiseptic swab; allow the site to dry.
- With the side of your nondominant hand, displace the skin away from the injection site, about 2.5 to 3.5 cm (1 to 1.5 in.).
- Hold the syringe like a dart and briskly insert the needle at a 90° angle to the skin surface. Insert fully.
- Stabilize the syringe with the thumb and forefinger of your nondominant hand. Keep displacing the skin with your other three fingers.
- **Be Safe!** Aspirate before injecting.
- Press the plunger at a 90° angle and slowly to inject the medication.
- Wait for 10 seconds; then remove the needle smoothly along the line of insertion. Release the skin.
- Engage the safety needle device, and dispose of supplies in a biohazard container.
- Gently blot the site with a gauze pad, and apply an adhesive bandage as needed.

Documentation

- Record scheduled medications on the MAR.
- Record PRN medications, including the reason given and response.
- Record medication, time, dose, and route given.
- Document therapeutic and adverse drug effects, nursing interventions, and teaching.
- Document assessment data before, during, and after injection (e.g., pain, bruising, or bleeding at the site).

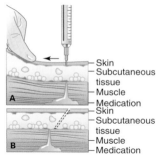

- Skin
- Subcutaneous tissue
- Muscle
- Medication

A

- Skin
- Subcutaneous tissue
- Muscle
- Medication

B

Displacing the skin and subcutaneous tissue over the muscle.

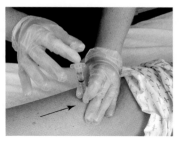

Giving an IM injection while stabilizing the syringe.

IV Infusions

Wilkinson Procedure 23-9E. Using a Prefilled Cartridge and Single-Dose Vial for IV Administration

✍ For steps to follow in all procedures, refer to the first page of this book, Universal Steps to follow in all Procedures. When administering medication, also follow the guidelines in Medication Guidelines: Steps to follow for All Medications in Tab 8 of this book.

Equipment

- Medication-prefilled cartridge.
- Alcohol prep pad or CHG-alcohol product.
- Syringe of the appropriate size for medication volume and viscosity.
- Filter needle.
- Safety needle.

Assessment

- Check that prefilled syringe is intact, and that the medication is clear, with no discoloration, cloudiness, or particles.

Post-Procedure Reassessment

- Assess for a change in color, cloudiness, particles in the medication mixed.

Key Points

- Be Smart! Before beginning, determine whether that volume is appropriate for the administration site.
- Maintain the sterility of the needle and medication.
- Assemble the prefilled cartridge and holder according to manufacturer's directions.
- Remove the needle cap from the prefilled cartridge, and set it on a sterile alcohol pad.
- Hold the cartridge vertically to expel the air and measure the correct dose of medication. Withdraw an amount of air equal to the volume of medication you need from the vial.
- Hold the cartridge with needle straight and insert the needle into the inverted vial, tip of the needle in the air above the medication (not in the fluid); inject the air into the vial. Be careful not to eject any medication from the cartridge into the vial.
- While maintaining pressure on the plunger, withdraw the ordered amount of vial medication, being careful not to withdraw any excess.

- Withdraw the needle or vial access device from the vial at a 90° angle and recap the needle.
- **Be Safe!** Always recap a sterile needle using a safety capping device or the one-handed scoop method.

Documentation
- Document per MAR, according to agency policy.

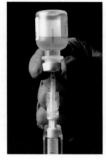

Injecting air into the vial makes the medication easier to withdraw.

Wilkinson Procedure 23-15. Adding Medication to an IV Infusion

✅ For steps to follow in all procedures, refer to the first page of this book, Universal Steps for All Procedures. When administering medication, also follow the guidelines in Medication Guidelines: Steps to follow for All Medications in Tab 8 of this book.

Equipment
- Prescribed IV solution.
- Syringe for medication.
- Needleless access device or safety needle (if a VAD is not available).
- Alcohol or CHG-alcohol prep pad.
- Label with medication, dose, date, time, and your initials.

Assessment
- Assess the patency and appearance of the IV site.
- **Be Safe!** Check the medication insert or drug formulary for appropriate time or rate for infusion and for preparation.

Post-Procedure Reassessment
- Check the IV line at least once every hour to ensure that the ordered or calculated rate is maintained.
- Assess the patient for complaints of pain at the infusion site.

Key Points
- Check the compatibility of the IV solution and medication.
- Refer to agency policy regarding maximum number of medications that can be added to one IV solution.
- Remove any protective covers, and inspect the bag or bottle for leaks, tears, or cracks. Inspect the fluid for clarity, color, and presence of particulate matter.
- Scrub all surfaces of the IV additive port with an alcohol or CHG-alcohol combination product.
- Check the expiration date.
- Assess the patency of the IV site.
- Maintain the sterility of IV fluids and medication admixture.
- Mix the IV solution and medication by gently turning the bag from end to end.
- **Be Smart!** Affix the medication label to the bag; include the medication name, dose, route, and your name. Be sure the label does not cover the solution label or volume marks.

Documentation

- If you added medication to an existing IV setup, document related patient assessment findings, such as appearance of IV site and complaints of pain or discomfort during administration.
- Findings are usually documented on an IV flow record rather than in the nursing notes.
- Added medications are sometimes charted on the MAR.
- Chart a nursing note only if there is something outside of the expected findings (e.g., if the IV has infiltrated).

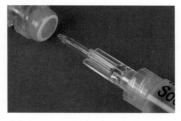

Inserting the needleless access device into the injection port.

Wilkinson Procedure 23-16A. Adding IV Push Medications Through an Infusing Primary IV Line

For steps to follow in all procedures, refer to the first page of this book, Universal Steps for All Procedures. When administering medication, also follow the guidelines in Medication Guidelines: Steps to follow for All Medications in Tab 8 of this book.

Equipment
- Syringe appropriate for medication volume and the type of line (e.g., peripheral IV, PICC, etc.)
- Alcohol prep pad, or CHG-alcohol combination product and gauze pad.
- Procedure gloves.
- If you are administering through an intermittent device:
  - Two 5- to 10-mL syringes, or one 10-mL syringe with 2 to 10 mL of normal saline for flushing the line, depending on site and facility policy.
  - One 5- to 10-mL syringe containing 2 to 5 mL of heparin flush (or saline) solution.

Assessment
- Be Safe! Assess the patency of the IV line before infusing.

Post-Procedure Reassessment
- Assess for complaints of pain or discomfort at the site.
- Check the site for redness, swelling, tenderness, and other signs of infiltration or phlebitis.

Key Points
- Be Smart! Determine the type and amount of dilution needed for the medication.
- Determine the amount of time needed to administer medication.
- Be Safe! Check the compatibility of the medication with the existing IV solution, if it is infusing.
- Ensure the patency of the line before administration.
- Prepare the medication from a vial or ampule or obtain the prescribed unit dose and verify medication with the order. Dilute as needed. Temporarily pause the infusion pump to administer the medication.
- Thoroughly scrub all surfaces of the injection port closest to the patient with the alcohol prep pad or CHG-alcohol combination product. Use povidone-iodine solution (Betadine) only if the patient is sensitive to the other products.

- Gently aspirate by slowly pulling back on the plunger to check for a blood return.
- Flush the line before and after administering the medication.
- If blood is returned (line is patent), pinch or clamp the IV tubing between the IV bag and the port, and slowly administer the rest of the medication.
- If the IV is patent (e.g., positive blood return), administer a small increment of the medication while observing for reactions to the medication.
- **Be Safe!** Maintain sterility.

Documentation

- Document related patient assessment findings, such as the appearance of the IV site and patient complaints of pain or discomfort during IV administration.
- You will usually document on an IV flow record and/or MAR rather than in the nursing notes.
- Chart a nursing note only if there is a problem (e.g., if the patient experiences pain when you administer the medication).

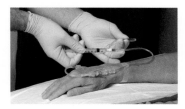

Giving IV push medication through a primary line.

Wilkinson Procedure 23-16C. Administering IV Push Through an IV Lock with IV Extension Tubing

For steps to follow in all procedures, refer to the first page of this book, Universal Steps for All Procedures. When administering medication, also follow the guidelines in Medication Guidelines: Steps to follow for All Medications in Tab 8 of this book.

Equipment

- Correct-size syringe for measuring medication.
- Needleless access cannula or safety needle.
- Antimicrobial swabs.
- IV extension set.
- Labels for the IV tubing and medication administration system.

Assessment

- Check the site for redness, swelling, tenderness, and other signs of infiltration or phlebitis.
- Perform assessments for evaluating the drug's effectiveness, such as checking BP after administering an antihypertensive agent.

Post-Procedure Reassessment

- Assess for patient complaints of pain or discomfort at the site.

Key Points

- Be Safe! Ensure the compatibility of the IV solution and medications.
- Be Smart! Calculate the amount of medication to administer.
- Be Safe! Use the correct rate of administration.
- Determine the volume of extension tubing attached to the access port.
- Assess the IV site and the patency of the line.
- Determine the correct primary line port for infusion of medication.
- Vigorously scrub all surfaces of the injection port closest to the patient with an antiseptic wipe.
- Administer a small amount of the flush solution and monitor for ease of administration, swelling at the IV site, or patient complaint of discomfort at the site.
- Again scrub the port.
- Use a slow, steady injection technique to administer the medication.
- Be Safe! If you feel resistance when flushing the line, look for a closed clamp on the catheter or tubing or clogged inline filter. Do not proceed until you are sure the catheter is correctly positioned and unobstructed.

- Remove the medication syringe.
- Vigorously scrub all surfaces of the injection connector for at least 15 seconds; then attach the flush syringe.
- Use a slow, steady injection technique when flushing the line.

Documentation

- Document related patient assessment findings, such as the appearance of the IV site and patient complaints of pain or discomfort during IV administration.
- You will usually document on an IV flow record and/or MAR rather than in the nursing notes.
- Chart a nursing note only if there is a problem (e.g., if the patient experiences pain when you administer the medication).

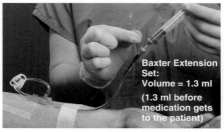

Baxter Extension Set:
Volume = 1.3 ml

(1.3 ml before medication gets to the patient)

Using slow, steady injection technique through an extension set.

Wilkinson Procedure 23-17A. Administering Medication by Intermittent Infusion Using a Volume-Control Administration Set

✓ For steps to follow in all procedures, refer to the first page of this book, Universal Steps for All Procedures. When administering medication, also follow the guidelines in Medication Guidelines: Steps to follow for All Medications in Tab 8 of this book.

Equipment
- Correct-size syringe for measuring medication.
- Needleless access cannula or safety needle.
- Small bag of diluted medication with piggyback tubing.
- Primary IV solution and tubing (unless one is already infusing).
- Antimicrobial swabs.
- Labels for the IV tubing and medication administration system.

Assessment
- Check the site for redness, swelling, tenderness, and other signs of infiltration or phlebitis.

Post-Procedure Reassessment
- Assess for complaints of pain or discomfort at the site.
  - Be Smart! Intermittent infusions are generally administered over 15 to 60 minutes, so you need to assess the patient as soon as the infusion begins and every 15 to 20 minutes until it is absorbed.
- Assess for factors that will provide a basis for evaluating the drug's effectiveness, such as checking BP after administering an antihypertensive agent.

Key Points
- Be Safe! Ensure the compatibility of the IV solution and medication.
- Be Smart! Be sure you have the correct tubing.
- Be Smart! Calculate the amount of medication to add to the solution.
- Use the correct amount and type of diluent solution.
- Be Safe! Use the correct rate of administration.
- Close both the upper and lower clamps on the tubing.
- Open the clamp of the air vent on the volume-control chamber.
- Maintaining sterile procedure, attach administration spike of the volume-control set to the primary IV bag.

- Fill the volume-control chamber with the desired amount of IV solution; then close the clamp.
- Prime the rest of the tubing.
- Scrub all surfaces of the injection port closest to the patient using an antiseptic swab.
- Connect the volume-control tubing to the extension tubing.
- Scrub the injection port on the volume-control chamber; attach the medication syringe using a blunt, needleless device; and inject the medication into the solution in the chamber.
- Gently rotate the chamber to mix the medication in the IV solution.
- Open the lower clamp, and start the infusion at the correct flow rate.
- **Be Safe!** Affix the correct label to the secondary bag, identifying the infusate, patient name, start date and hour, discard date and hour, and your initials.

Documentation
- Record the appearance of the IV site and patient complaints of pain or discomfort during IV administration.
- You will usually document on an IV flow record and/or MAR rather than in the nursing notes.
- Chart a nursing note only if there is a problem (e.g., if the patient experiences pain when you administer the medication).

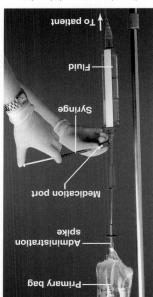

To patient ↑

Fluid

Syringe

Medication port

Administration
spike

Primary bag

Adding medication to the volume-control chamber.

Wilkinson Procedure 23-17B. Administering Medication by Intermittent Infusion (Piggyback Set)

For steps to follow in all procedures, refer to the first page of this book, Universal Steps for All Procedures. When administering medication, also follow the guidelines in Medication Guidelines: Steps to follow for All Medications in Tab 8 of this book.

Equipment
- Correct-size syringe for measuring medication.
- Needleless access cannula or safety needle.
- Small bag of diluted medication with piggyback tubing.
- Primary IV solution and tubing (unless one is already infusing).
- Antimicrobial swabs.
- Labels for the IV tubing and medication administration system.

Assessment
- Check the site for redness, swelling, tenderness, and other signs of infiltration or phlebitis.

Post-Procedure Reassessment
- Assess for complaints of pain or discomfort at the site.
  - Be Smart! Intermittent infusions are generally administered over 15 to 60 minutes, so you need to assess the patient as soon as the infusion begins and every 15 to 20 minutes until it is absorbed.
- Assess for factors that will provide a basis for evaluating the drug's effectiveness, such as checking BP after administering an antihypertensive agent.

Key Points
- Be Safe! Ensure the compatibility of the IV solution and medication, in both the primary and secondary (piggyback) systems.
- Be Smart! Be sure you have the correct tubing. Piggyback tubing is short; tandem tubing is long.
- Be Smart! Calculate the amount of medication to add to the solution. Use the correct amount and type of diluent solution.
- Be Safe! Use the correct rate of administration.
- Be sure the slide clamp is closed. Squeeze the drip chamber, filling it one-third to one-half full.

- Open the clamp and prime the tubing, holding the end of the tubing lower than the bag of fluid.
- **Be Safe!** Affix the correct label to the piggyback bag, identifying the infusate, patient name, start date and hour, discard date and hour, and your initials.
- Hang the piggyback container on the IV pole. Lower the primary IV container to hang below the level of the piggyback IV.
- Open the clamp of the piggyback line and regulate to the prescribed infusion rate for the medication.
- At the end of the infusion, clamp the piggyback tubing, and reset the primary bag to its correct infusion rate.

Documentation

- Record the appearance of the IV site and patient complaints of pain or discomfort during IV administration.
- You will usually document on an IV flow record and/or MAR rather than in the nursing notes.
- Chart a nursing note only if there is a problem (e.g., if the patient experiences pain when you administer the medication).

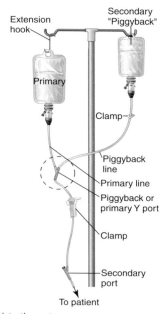

Piggyback administration set.

Wilkinson Procedure 23-18. Administering Medication through a Central Venous Access Device

✔️ For steps to follow in all procedures, refer to the first page of this book, Universal Steps for All Procedures. When administering medication, also follow the guidelines in Medication Guidelines: Steps to follow for All Medications in Tab 8 of this book.

Equipment
- Syringe appropriate for medication volume; needleless device or safety syringe with a filter needle for drawing up the medication.
- 2 syringes for the flush solution.
- Saline or heparin flush solution, as prescribed.
- Alcohol prep pad or CHG-alcohol combination product and gauze pad.
- Procedure gloves.

Assessment
- Carefully palpate the area around the insertion site through the dressing.
- If the patient has tenderness, assess further for other signs of complications.
- Visually assess the surrounding catheter insertion site for redness, swelling, warmth, or drainage.

Post-Procedure Reassessment
- Monitor for signs of:
  - Catheter complications (e.g., shortness of breath, chest pain, engorged veins at the surface of the skin, and palpitations).
  - Catheter dislodgment (e.g., neck swelling or pain, bleeding at the site or within the line, palpitations, or gurgling noise or the sound of running water on the side of the catheter insertion).
- Look for difficulty moving the neck or jaw, headache, or ear pain.
- Assess for signs of:
  - Catheter-related infection (e.g., fever, increased WBC count, redness, warmth at the site).
  - Leaking or blood backup at the injection ports, tubing connections, and the site.
- Observe for bleeding at the CVAD site.
- Assess for allergic response or adverse effects to medication.
- Conduct a comprehensive pain assessment.

Key Points

- **Be Safe!** First verify the medication can be administered safely through a central site.
- **Be Safe!** Be sure you've are using the correct port.
- Scrub all surfaces of the catheter port, including the extension "leg," with an alcohol or CHG-alcohol combination product every time you access the line.
- Flush the line before and after administering medication. Use saline, heparinized flush solution, or solution from the infusing IV line.
- Clamp the line between the IV infusion set and the medication port. Open the clamp after medication is administered.
- After administration, monitor and report suspected CVAD dislodgment, line-related infection, or other complications.

Documentation

- Record signs of:
    - Allergic response to or adverse effects of medication.
    - Catheter complications, catheter dislodgment, or catheter-related infection.
- Record the date and time tubing and port cap are changed.
- Document all medications infused through the CVAD—usually on a flowsheet and/or a MAR.

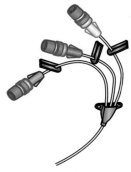

Multilumen central venous access device.

Wilkinson Procedure 36-1. Initiating a Peripheral IV Infusion

✔️ For steps to follow in all procedures, refer to the first page of this book, Universal Steps for All Procedures. When administering medication, also follow the guidelines in Medication Guidelines: Steps to follow for All Medications in Tab 8 of this book.

Equipment
- IV solution.
- Administration set or IV lock and injection caps.
- IV catheter.
- If using extension tubing, a saline-filled syringe to prime it.
- Procedure gloves.
- Scissors.
- Antiseptic swabs containing CHG or 70% alcohol wipes.
- Tourniquet (nonlatex, if available).
- Sterile catheter stabilization device or ½-in. tape; 2 in. × 2 in. sterile gauze and/or transparent semipermeable occlusive dressing.
- 1-in. hypoallergenic tape, preferably clear.
- Labels, time tape.
- Linen-saver pad.
- Arm board, if necessary.
- Be Smart! For a glass solution container, use vented tubing; for a plastic container, you may use either vented or nonvented tubing.

Assessment
- Check VS, laboratory values, urine output, skin turgor, breath sounds, and the condition of mucous membranes to confirm the need for IV therapy.
- Assess the veins on the arms and hands for a potential insertion site.
- Assess for allergy to tape and check the medical record for complicating factors such as anticoagulant therapy, bleeding disorders, or low platelet count.

Post-Procedure Reassessment
- Monitor the IV site and flow rate (many agency standards require hourly), as well as signs of infiltration, inflammation, and phlebitis.
- Monitor tolerance of IV therapy: auscultate lungs and monitor VS, I&O, laboratory values, and neck vein distention.

- **Be Safe!** Report signs of fluid overload, such as:
  - Crackles.
  - Edema.
  - Shortness of breath.
  - Diminished urine output.
  - Increased BP.
  - Increased heart rate with bounding pulse.
  - Distended neck veins.

Key Points

- Prepare the IV solution and administration set, including extension tubing and volume control device if used.
- Apply the tourniquet.
- **Be Safe!** Keep the catheter sterile throughout the procedure.
- **Be Smart!** Locate a vein. As a rule, select the most distal vein in an upper extremity.
- Don clean nonsterile gloves and cleanse the site. Allow the antiseptic to dry on the skin. Do not touch the site after cleansing.
- Use your nondominant hand to apply gentle traction on skin at the insertion site to stabilize the vein.
- Inform the patient that you are about to insert the catheter.
- Hold the catheter, bevel up, at a 30° to 45° angle and pierce the skin.
- Lower the catheter so it is parallel to the skin, and advance it.
- Watch for a flashback of blood; continue inserting the catheter. Advance the catheter halfway, then remove (or retract) the needle as you insert the catheter the rest of the way—to the hub.
- While holding the catheter in place with one hand, release the tourniquet with your other hand.
- Connect the IV administration set or extension tubing to the IV catheter.
- Adjust the flow rate according to the prescriber's order.
- Secure the connection, stabilize the catheter, and apply dressing to the IV insertion site.
- Secure the tubing by looping and taping it to the skin.
- Label the dressing, tubing, and IV solution. Apply a time tape.
- Place an arm board as needed.

Documentation
- Record the date and time of insertion, gauge and type of catheter, number of attempts, and location of the insertion site.
- State whether you used a tourniquet, blood returned in the catheter, the IV was flushed, and the type and amount of flush solution used.
- Describe the dressing and tape type used, the method of stabilizing the IV line, and the type and rate of the IV fluid infusing.
- Describe patient's tolerance of the procedure, any adverse reactions, teaching done, and any interventions that were required.
- Often, IV care is documented on a flowsheet.
- Document on the I&O sheet the amounts of fluids infused.

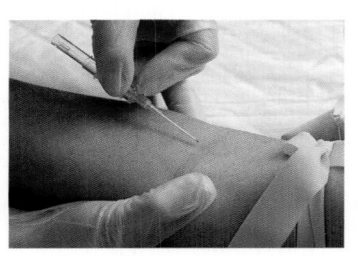

Pierce the skin at a 30° to 45° angle.

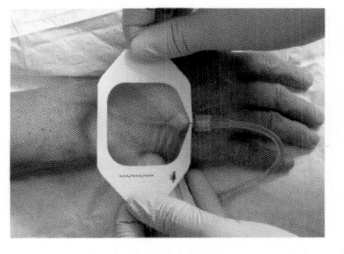

Secure the IV catheter at the hub with transparent dressing.

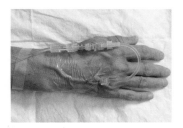

Smooth the transparent dressing to the skin.

Wilkinson Procedure 36-4B. Changing the IV Solution and Tubing

✔️ For steps to follow in all procedures, refer to the first page of this book, Universal Steps for All Procedures.

Equipment
- Nonsterile gloves.
- Administration set.
- IV solution.
- IV pole.
- Antiseptic swabs that contain solutions such as alcohol or CHG.
  - Be Safe! CHG is not recommended for infants younger than age 2 months.
- 1-in. nonallergenic tape.
- Time tape.
- Watch with a second hand or digital readout.

Assessment
- Check the IV catheter insertion date (the CDC recommends changing a peripheral IV every 72 to 96 hours).
- Assess the IV catheter for patency.
- Assess the IV site for signs of phlebitis, infiltration, infection, or inflammation.
- Be Safe! If any of these complications exist, discontinue the current IV and start a new one.

Post-Procedure Reassessment
- Be Safe! Evaluate proper IV rate regularly (usually hourly). Continue to monitor the insertion site for signs of infiltration, inflammation, infection, and phlebitis.
- Evaluate the effectiveness of IV therapy by assessing hydration status or expected effect of the IV medication/solution.

Key Points
- Be Safe! Care of IVs requires careful sterile technique.
- Prepare and hang the new IV solution and tubing.
- Close the roller clamp on the administration set.
- Wearing clean nonsterile gloves, place a sterile swab under the catheter hub.

- Remove the protective cover from the distal end of the new administration set.
- Stabilize the IV catheter while applying pressure over the vein just above the insertion site.
- Disengage the old tubing from the IV catheter and insert the new tubing.
- Be Smart! If the tubing does not separate, use a hemostat to twist the lock. Grip and twist lightly.
- Adjust the drip rate or set and turn on the volume control pump.
- Cleanse the IV site, resecure the IV catheter and tubing connection; loop and tape the tubing.
- Label tubing and solution with date, initials, rate, and time tape.

Documentation

- Fluid and tubing changes are usually documented on a flowsheet.
- If writing a nursing note, document:
    - The date and time the IV fluid and tubing were changed.
    - Type of IV fluid and rate of infusion.
    - The location and condition of the IV catheter insertion site.
    - Any complications of IV therapy and the interventions taken.

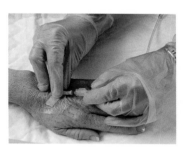

Stabilize the catheter and apply pressure over the vein while disconnecting the administration set.

Wilkinson Procedure 36-5B. Changing IV Dressings (Central Line Dressings)

✔ For steps to follow in all procedures, refer to the first page of this book, Universal Steps for All Procedures.

Equipment
- Clean nonsterile gloves.
- Central line dressing kit (including sterile gloves, mask, sterile transparent semipermeable dressing, sterile tape, an antimicrobial agent, and a sterile catheter stabilization device).
- Mask for patient.
- A sponge containing the antimicrobial agent CHG may be used as a part of the dressing, as well.
  - **Note:** You can use povidone-iodine followed by alcohol as the antimicrobial if CHG is contraindicated and if the patient is not allergic to iodine.

Assessment
- Observe the site for excessive bleeding, infection, or other complications.
- Observe for signs of compromised catheter integrity: wet dressing, kinked, cracked, or leaking catheter.
- Be Safe! Notify the primary provider if any of these signs are present.

Post-Procedure Reassessment
- Evaluate the IV insertion site and surrounding tissue for signs of infiltration, inflammation, infection, and phlebitis.
- Monitor the dressing for dampness, blood, soiling, or loosening.
- Continue to visually inspect and palpate the catheter-skin junction site for tenderness daily through the transparent dressing.

Key Points
- Be Safe! Care of CVCs requires meticulous aseptic technique.
- Obtain sterile central line dressing kit and mask for the patient. If there is no kit, you will need at least a mask, sterile gloves, antiseptic solution, dressing, and tape.
- Place the patient in a comfortable position. Some guidelines advise semi-Fowler's.
- Ask the patient to don a mask or turn his head to the opposite side if unable to tolerate a mask.

- Don mask and clean nonsterile gloves.
- Carefully remove the old dressing and stabilization device.
- Inspect the site for signs of complications.
- Remove and discard gloves and soiled dressing; wash your hands.
- Don sterile gloves contained in the kit.
- Scrub the site for 30 seconds, using swabs contained in the kit.
- Scrub the sutures (if any) and the catheter, from insertion site to the hub or bifurcation.
- Allow the site to dry.
- Apply the dressing that comes in the kit.
- Apply the new catheter stabilization device, if one is used.
- Remove the drape, if one was used.
- Loop the catheter gently and secure it with tape to the skin. Avoid securing it to the dressing.
- Label the dressing with the date changed, time, and your initials.

Documentation

- Chart the date and time the dressing was changed, and condition of the IV catheter insertion site.
- Document any complications of IV therapy and the interventions taken. Document the dressing change on the IV record.
- Often, IV care is documented on a flowsheet.

Wilkinson Procedure 36-6. Converting a Primary Line to a Heparin or Saline Lock

✅ For steps to follow in all procedures, refer to the first page of this book, Universal Steps for All Procedures.

Equipment
- Clean nonsterile gloves.
- Peripheral intermittent lock adapter.
- 2 syringes containing saline or dilute heparin solution.
- Linen-saver pad.
- Transparent semipermeable dressing.
- Alcohol or other antiseptic swab.

Assessment
- Assess the patient's readiness to have the IV fluid discontinued and the site changed to an intermittent lock (e.g., tolerating oral fluids, adequate urine output, and laboratory values within normal limits).
- Assess for allergy to tape.
- Assess the IV site for signs of phlebitis, infiltration, extravasation, or infection.

Post-Procedure Reassessment
- Evaluate catheter patency before each use and routinely every 8 to 24 hours (according to agency policy).
- Monitor the insertion site for signs of complications, and the patient's tolerance to the intermittent IV therapy.

Key Points
- Be Safe! If complications are present or the IV has been in place longer than 72 to 96 hours, remove the IV catheter instead of converting it to an intermittent lock.
- Don clean nonsterile gloves.
- Remove the IV lock from the package, and flush the adapter.
- Remove the IV dressing and the tape that is securing the tubing.
- Close the roller clamp on the administration set.
- With your nondominant hand, apply pressure over the vein just above the insertion site; stabilize the catheter hub with your thumb and forefinger.

- Disengage the old tubing from the IV catheter.
- **Be Smart!** If the tubing does not separate from the catheter, use a hemostat to gently twist the lock and separate tubing from catheter.
- Quickly insert the lock adapter into the IV catheter and turn the lock adapter until snug.
- Scrub the adapter injection port for at least 15 seconds.
- Flush the lock adapter again.
- Apply a sterile transparent semipermeable dressing.
- **Be Safe!** Do not cover the lock-hub connection.
- Label the dressing with the date and your initials.
- Discard used supplies.
- **Be Safe!** Maintain sterility of equipment throughout.

Documentation
- Chart the date and time the IV line was converted to an intermittent lock device; the size and location of the catheter; and the type and amount of flush solution used.
- Document the condition of the IV site and any signs of complications.
- Record on the I&O record the amount of IV fluid infused.
- Often, IV care is documented on a flowsheet or an electronic patient record.

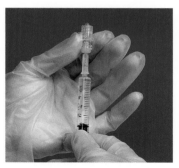

Flush the adapter.

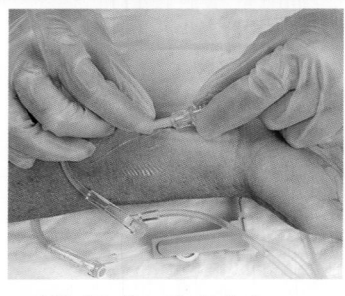

Insert the adapter quickly into the catheter hub.

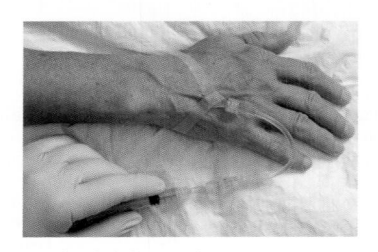

Flush the line again after it is inserted.

Wilkinson Procedure 36-7. Discontinuing a Peripheral IV

For steps to follow in all procedures, refer to the first page of this book, Universal Steps for All Procedures.

Equipment
- Clean nonsterile gloves, sterile 2 in. × 2 in. gauze dressings.
- 1-in. tape or transparent semipermeable dressing.
- Linen-saver pad.

Assessment
- Verify the order and assess the patient's readiness to have the IV fluid discontinued (e.g., tolerating oral fluids, has adequate urine output, laboratory values are within normal limits).

Post-Procedure Reassessment
- Assess the integrity of the removed catheter; compare the length to the original insertion length to ensure the entire catheter is removed.
  - Be Smart! If a catheter defect is noted, report to the manufacturer and regulatory agencies and complete an incident report according to agency policy.
- Monitor the patient's response to oral fluids after IV therapy is discontinued. Note changes in the patient's condition that might indicate the need to re-establish IV therapy.

Key Points
- Be Smart! Place a linen-saver pad under the extremity with the IV catheter to prevent soiling patient's clothing or bed linen.
- Don clean nonsterile gloves, and close the roller clamp on the administration set.
- Carefully remove the IV dressing, catheter stabilizer, and tape securing the tubing.
- Scrub the catheter-skin junction with an antiseptic pad.
- Place a sterile 2 in. × 2 in. gauze pad above the IV insertion site and gently remove the catheter. Do not press on the gauze pad while removing the catheter.
- Be Safe! Apply firm pressure with the gauze pad over the insertion site. Hold pressure for 1 to 3 minutes; hold longer if bleeding persists.
- Apply a folded sterile 2 in. × 2 in. gauze pad. Secure it with tape.

Documentation
- You will usually record this procedure on a flowsheet or in the electronic patient record.
- Chart the date and time IV therapy was discontinued.
- Note the condition of the site, including the presence of any complications.
- If complications are present, document your interventions and notify the primary care provider.

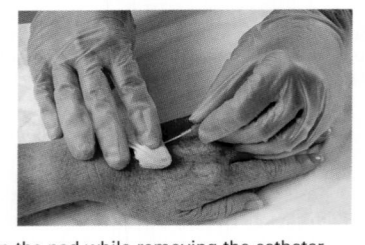

Do not press on the pad while removing the catheter.

Wilkinson Procedure 36-8A. Administering Blood and Blood Products

For steps to follow in all procedures, refer to the first page of this book, Universal Steps for All Procedures. When administering medication, also follow the guidelines in Medication Guidelines: Steps to follow for All Medications in Tab 8 of this book.

Equipment
- Clean nonsterile gloves.
- Blood product.
- 250 mL normal saline IV solution.
- Blood administration set with a 200-micrometer filter and Luer-Lok connection (if there is no filter on the tubing, you must attach one).
  - Be Smart! Although nurses commonly use a 20-gauge catheter, for routine transfusion, a 22- or 24-gauge can be used. You would need an 18- or 20-gauge catheter to transfuse large amounts of blood rapidly.
  - Be Smart! When choosing an IV catheter for transfusion, the primary consideration should be the size of the patient's veins and not an arbitrary catheter size.
- IV pole.
- Watch with a second hand or digital readout.
- Thermometer.
- BP cuff with sphygmomanometer.
- Stethoscope.

Assessment
- Confirm the patient's need for blood products by assessing VS, urine output, and laboratory studies.
- Be Safe! Check the history for previous transfusions and reactions. Verify the patient's blood type.
- Assess that the existing IV catheter is patent and the proper size for blood product administration.
- Assess the IV insertion site for signs of infiltration, phlebitis, infection, or inflammation.
- Assess for allergy to tape.

Post-Procedure Reassessment

■ Be Safe! Monitor for signs of fluid overload and for signs and symptoms of transfusion reaction.

■ Check laboratory studies, such as complete blood count, to help evaluate the effectiveness of therapy and identify transfusion reaction.

Key Points

■ Verify that informed consent has been obtained.

■ Verify the prescriber's order, noting the indication, and rate of infusion.

■ Administer any prescribed pretransfusion medications.

■ Obtain a blood administration set and 250 mL of IV normal saline solution.

■ Obtain the blood product from the blood bank according to your institution's policy.

■ With another qualified staff member, and using two identifiers, verify the patient and blood product identification (e.g., birth date, hospital ID number, blood type).

■ Be Safe! Contact the blood bank immediately if there are discrepancies, and do not administer the blood product.

■ Document on the blood bank form the date and time the transfusion is begun.

■ Check that all clamps are closed on the blood administration set; label the tubing.

■ Hang the normal saline and prime the tubing.

■ Gently invert the blood product container several times.

■ Spike the blood product and hang the blood on the IV pole.

■ Obtain a set of VS.

■ Scrub the port with an alcohol or CHG-alcohol antiseptic swab for at least 15 seconds

■ Attach the administration set tubing to the IV catheter.

■ Slowly open the roller clamp closest to the blood product.

■ Be Safe! Infuse the first 50 mL slowly and remain with the patient for the first 5 minutes.

■ Measure VS at 5 minutes, 15 minutes, and 30 minutes; then hourly.

■ Observe for and ask the patient to report symptoms of transfusion reaction.

■ When the blood has transfused, flush the line with the saline solution.

■ Disconnect the tubing from the IV catheter, and dispose of the blood product container and tubing per agency policy.

- If a second unit of blood is to be transfused, the same administration set may be used.
- Administer any post-transfusion medications prescribed.

Documentation
- Chart the date, time, and reason the transfusion was started.
- Document transfusion VS according to institution policy (many institutions have a special form for this).
- Record the amount of blood transfused on the I&O record.
- Chart any complications and the interventions taken.

Wilkinson Procedure 36-9. Assisting with Percutaneous Central Venous Catheter Placement

For steps to follow in all procedures, refer to the first page of this book, Universal Steps for All Procedures.

Equipment
- Sterile gloves (2 or 3 pairs).
- Masks, hats, barrier gowns.
- 10-mL vials of normal saline (3 or 4), 2 or 3 syringes with 1-in. needle.
- 25-gauge ⅝-in., and 18-gauge 1½-in. needles (2 or 3 of each).
- CVC kit containing: an introducer, antiseptic solution/swabs, sterile drapes, 10-mL syringe, 1% or 2% Xylocaine without epinephrine, suture, sterile scissors, and needle holder.
- CVC (single-lumen or multilumen).
- Injection caps.
- Alcohol wipes.

Assessment
- Obtain baseline VS.
- Verify that informed consent has been given.
- Assess for allergy to tape.

Post-Procedure Reassessment
- Be Safe! Obtain VS.
- Ausculate the lungs and assess for respiratory distress, sharp chest pain, and coughing.
- Monitor for 24 hours for these signs.
- Assess the patient daily to determine continuing need for the CVC.

Key Points
- Be Safe! Perform meticulous hand hygiene.
- Be Safe! Use gowns and maximum barrier precautions.
- Be Safe! Use meticulous sterile technique.
- Obtain VS and verify informed consent.
- Gather and set up supplies and equipment.
- Prepare sterile field, and add supplies.
- Position the patient (Trendelenburg with a rolled towel between the shoulders).

- Offer mask, gown, and sterile gloves to physician.
- Don sterile gloves and mask (or follow agency policy).
- Prep an 8 × 10-in. area around the site, using applicators of 2% CHG in 70% alcohol, per agency guidelines.
- Place the large sterile drape to cover patient's head and chest.
- Have the patient turn his head opposite the direction of insertion.
- Observe while the physician inserts and sutures the catheter.
- Apply sterile transparent dressing, close any lumen clamps, and place tape across the lumens near the injection caps.
- Monitor for complications (especially respiratory distress).
- Be Safe! Obtain a chest x-ray to confirm correct placement of the catheter tip.

Documentation
- Document date and time of catheter insertion, catheter type and size, and site location.
- Chart:
  - Assessments and interventions performed at insertion and immediately after.
  - Patient's tolerance of procedure (subjective and objective data).
  - X-ray verification of catheter placement.

Nutrition

Wilkinson Procedure 26-1. Checking Fingerstick (Capillary) Blood Glucose Levels

✔ For steps to follow in all procedures, refer to the first page of this book, Universal Steps for All Procedures.

Equipment
- Blood glucose meter; test strip.
- Sterile lancet (and injector, if available).
- Alcohol or other antiseptic pad, if required by agency policy.
- 2 in. × 2 in. gauze pad or cotton ball.
- Procedure gloves.

Assessment
- Assess the patient's understanding of the procedure.
- Check for factors such as anticoagulant therapy or low platelet count.
- Assess potential puncture sites for bruising, inflammation, lesions, poor circulation, or edema.
  - Be Safe! Avoid such sites because of risk for infection and inaccurate results.

Post-Procedure Reassessment
- Assess the puncture site for bleeding or bruising. Evaluate the patient's understanding of the procedure and the test results.
  - Be Smart! Notify the primary care provider of abnormal test results, or administer insulin based on test results, as prescribed.

Key Points
- Ask the patient to wash her hands with warm soap and water. Dry well with a clean towel.
- Don procedure gloves.
- Cleanse the patient's finger with an alcohol prep pad if agency policy requires.
- Prepare the lancet and meter and obtain a clean test strip that is recommended for the meter. Check the code on the container.
- Stick the side of the patient's fingertip.
- Be Safe! Use a different finger each time.

- Wipe off the first drop of blood; place the second drop on the test strip.
- At the indicated time, read the glucose level on the digital display. (Follow the manufacturer's instructions.)

Documentation

- Usually you will record the test result on a flowsheet.
- If the fingerstick is performed in response to patient symptoms, you may need to write a narrative note. Include:
  - Date and time the test was performed.
  - Whether you notified the primary care provider.
  - Any treatment given.
  - Patient teaching provided.

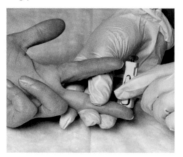

Position the injector firmly against the fingertip.

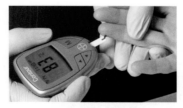

Place the second drop of blood on the test strip.

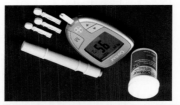

Read the result on the digital display.

Wilkinson Procedure 26-2. Inserting Nasogastric and Nasoenteric Tubes

✓ For steps to follow in all procedures, refer to the first page of this book, Universal Steps for All Procedures.

Equipment

- NG tube (commonly 16 or 18 Fr for adults) or NE (small bowel) tube (8, 10, or 12 Fr).
- Stylet or guidewire (for small-bore tubes), according to agency policy.
- Procedure gloves.
- Linen-saver pad or towel.
- Water-soluble lubricant.
- 50- to 60-mL catheter-tip syringe or bulb syringe for Salem sump tubes.
- 30-mL Luer-Lok syringe for small-bore feeding tubes.
- Hypoallergenic tape (2.5 cm [1 in.] wide) or tube fixation device.
- Indelible marker.
- Skin adhesive.
- Stethoscope.
- Basin of warm water (for plastic tube) or ice (for rubber tube).
- Glass of water with a straw; penlight; tongue blade; pH test strip.
- Tissues.
- Safety pin.
- Gauze square or small plastic bag.
- Rubber band.
- Suction equipment (if tube is being connected to suction).

Assessment

- Verify:
  - The medical prescription for type of tube and whether it is to be attached to suction or drainage.
  - The patient's need for NG or NE intubation (e.g., surgery involving the GI tract, impaired swallowing, or decreased level of consciousness).
- Check medical history for:
  - Anticoagulant therapy.
  - Coagulopathy.
  - Nasal trauma.
  - Nasal surgery.

■ Epistaxis.

■ Deviated septum.

■ Assess each naris for deviated septum and skin breakdown.

■ Ask the patient to close each nostril alternately and breathe; select the nostril with the greatest air flow.

■ Assess the level of consciousness and ability to follow instructions.

■ Ask the patient to blow her nose, if not contraindicated.

■ Be Safe! Assess for a gag reflex, using a tongue blade. Absence of gag reflex increases the risk for aspiration.

■ Be Smart! Contraindications to NG insertion by a nurse include:

   ■ Maxillofacial disorders, surgery, or trauma.

   ■ Esophageal tumors or surgery.

   ■ Laryngectomy.

   ■ Skull fracture.

   ■ Unstable high cervical spinal injuries.

   ■ Esophageal varices.

Post-Procedure Reassessment

■ Assess the patient's tolerance of the procedure (e.g., discomfort, gagging, coughing, respiratory status) and whether she is comfortable.

■ Note the color, consistency, and pH of NG or NE aspirate.

Key Points

■ Place the patient in a sitting or high-Fowler's position.

■ Measure the length of the tube.

   ■ NG tubes: Measure from tip of the nose to earlobe and from earlobe to xiphoid process.

   ■ NE tubes: Add 8 to 10 cm (3 to 4 in.) to the NG measurement, as directed.

■ Lubricate the tube with water-soluble lubricant.

■ Have the patient hyperextend her neck and breathe through her mouth.

■ Insert the tube gently through the nostril and advance the tube as the patient swallows.

■ Instruct the patient to tilt her head forward, drink water, and swallow.

■ Be Safe! Withdraw the tube immediately if respiratory distress occurs during or immediately after insertion.

- **Be Safe!** Confirm tube placement initially by x-ray. Always reconfirm tube placement with a combination of bedside methods before giving feedings or medicine.
- **Be Smart!** Secure the tube to the nose and to the patient's gown.

Documentation

- Chart:
  - Date and time of insertion.
  - Size and type of the NG or NE tube.
  - Insertion site (which naris).
  - Length of tube from tip of the nose to the end of the tube.
  - Tolerance of the procedure.
  - Any abnormal findings.
  - Methods for confirming tube placement.
  - Description of gastric contents.
  - Respiratory status.
- You will document NG or NE tube insertion in progress notes and flowsheets in most agencies.

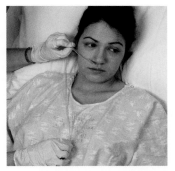

Measure from tip of nose to earlobe, then to the xiphoid process.

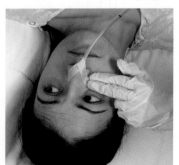

Apply tape to the patient's nose.

Wilkinson Procedure 26-3. Administering Feedings Through Gastric and Enteric Tubes

For steps to follow in all procedures, refer to the first page of this book, Universal Steps for All Procedures.

Equipment
- Prescribed feeding formula at room temperature.
- Filtered water or prescribed diluent, if ordered.
- Tube feeding administration set and bag.
- 60-mL Luer-Lok or catheter-tip syringe (2 needed for syringe feeding).
- Connector to connect administration set to the feeding tube.
- Stethoscope.
- IV pole.
- Linen-saver pad.
- Graduated container.
- pH strip.
- Enteral feeding infusion pump.
- *For gastrostomy and jejunostomy tubes:* a small precut gauze dressing.

Assessment
- Check patient history for food allergies.
- Check the length of the exposed tube.
  - Compare the length from the naris to the connector recorded after x-ray confirmation of placement.
  - Observe the mark that was made on it where it entered the nostril after insertion.
  - Be Safe! If there is significant change in length, tube position must again be confirmed by radiography.
- Assess fluid status by checking breath sounds, mucous membranes, skin turgor, edema, and I&O.
- Obtain baseline weight and laboratory studies.
- Monitor VS before and after feedings.
- Auscultate for bowel sounds before each feeding or every 4 to 8 hours for continuous feedings.
- Also check for distention, nausea, vomiting, and diarrhea.
- *For gastrostomy and jejunostomy tubes:* Assess the exit site at every shift. Report redness or drainage to the primary care provider.

Post-Procedure Reassessment

- Assess tolerance to the tube feeding (abdominal discomfort, nausea, vomiting, or diarrhea).
- Assess bowel sounds and VS every 4 hours.
- Check gastric residual volume every 4 hours.
- Monitor I&O every 8 hours.
- Weigh patient at least 3 times per week.
- Monitor the exit site for signs of skin breakdown.
- Assess frequency of bowel movements.
- Check laboratory values to evaluate nutritional status.

Key Points

- Check the medical prescription for the type of formula, rate, route, and frequency of feeding. Check the expiration date on the feeding.
- **Be Safe!** Check the chart to make sure there is a radiographic confirmation of tube placement.
- **Be Safe!** Confirm tube placement with a combination of bedside methods before administering the feeding. Bedside methods include:
  - Measuring pH of aspirate.
  - Changes in residual volume.
  - Observing the length of the exposed tube.
  - Injecting air into the tube and auscultating ("whoosh" test).
  - Asking the patient to speak.
- **Be Safe!** Elevate the head of the bed at least 30° to 45° while administering the feedings and for an hour after administration.
- Check residual volume before feeding for intermittent feedings.
  - *For continuous feeding:* Check gastric residual volume at least once every shift. If the residual is 10% greater than the formula flow rate for 1 hour (or > 150 mL), hold the feeding for 1 hour and recheck. Notify the primary provider if the residual is still not within normal limits.
  - *For gastrostomy and PEG tubes and gastrostomy buttons (G-buttons):* Check residual volume every 4 hours.
  - **Be Smart!** *For jejunostomy tubes:* Residual volumes are not checked.
- Flush tubing with 30 mL of water before and after feeding (every 4 hours for continuous feedings), and before and after medication administration.
- Label and hang the bag, prime the tubing and thread it through the pump, regulate the gravity drip rate, or elevate the syringe to feed with an open-system syringe.

- ■ **Be Smart!** Remember to unclamp the tubing!
- ■ Change the tube feeding administration set and other supplies a minimum of every 24 hours.
- ■ **Be Smart!** Continuous feedings should be infused by pump.

Documentation
- ■ Chart the type of tube feeding, rate and volume of infusion, amount of gastric residual volume (if any), and tolerance of procedure.
- ■ Document feeding amount on the I&O flowsheet.
- ■ Record all flushes as intake; subtract any liquids that you aspirate and do not reinstill (e.g., when gastric residual is too high).

Wilkinson Procedure 26-4. Removing a Nasogastric or Nasoenteric Tube

For steps to follow in all procedures, refer to the first page of this book, Universal Steps for All Procedures.

Equipment
- Linen-saver pad.
- 60-mL Luer-Lok or catheter-tip syringe.
- Procedure gloves.
- Stethoscope.
- Disposable plastic bag.
- Emesis basin.
- Gauze square.

Assessment
- To confirm readiness for discontinuing the NG or NE tube, auscultate the abdomen for the presence of bowel sounds and assess the patient's ability to consume an oral diet.
- Be Smart! Determine how long it has been since the last tube feeding, and wait at least 30 minutes to remove the feeding tube.

Post-Procedure Reassessment
- Assess the nares for signs of skin breakdown or bleeding.
- Monitor for signs of GI dysfunction, such as food intolerance, nausea, vomiting, and abdominal distention.
- Monitor bowel sounds.
- Monitor I&O every 8 hours.
- Weigh the patient regularly.
- Monitor laboratory values to evaluate nutritional status.

Key Points
- Verify the primary provider's order for removal of NG or NE tube.
- Assist the patient to a sitting or high-Fowler's position.
- Place the linen-saver pad on the patient's chest and don gloves.
- If the NG tube is connected to suction, turn it off.
- Stand on the patient's right side if you are right-handed; on the left side if left-handed.
- Inject 10 mL of air through the main lumen to clear the tube of secretions.

- Unpin the tube from the gown and remove the tape from the nose.
- Pinch the tube with one hand, hold gauze to the patient's nose with the other hand, ready to grab the tube upon removal.
- Ask the patient to hold his breath, and gently, but quickly, withdraw the tube and place it in the plastic bag.
- Discard the equipment.
- Provide or assist with care of the nose and mouth.

Documentation

- Chart:
  - Date and time of removal.
  - Patient's tolerance of the procedure.
  - The amount of drainage if the tube was connected to suction.
- Note any complications following tube removal (e.g., food intolerance, nausea, vomiting, and abdominal distention).

Wilkinson Procedure 26-5. Administering Parenteral Nutrition

✔️ For steps to follow in all procedures, refer to the first page of this book, Universal Steps for All Procedures.

Equipment
- PN solution.
- Procedure gloves.
- Sterile gloves (per agency policy and type of tubing connection).
- IV administration set, extension set if indicated.
- 0.22-micron filter (1.2-micron filter if solution contains albumin or lipids).
- Time tape.
- 70% alcohol pads or CHG-based pads.
- Infusion pump.
- 10-mL syringe and saline.
- Blood glucose testing monitor.
- I&O record.
- Transparent dressing or sterile gauze and tape (if dressing is to be changed).
  - If the dressing is to be changed, you also need a transparent dressing or sterile gauze, tape, and a mask.
- Catheter stabilization device.
  - **Be Smart!** A catheter stabilization device (e.g., StatLock) is recommended for all catheters and must be changed with each dressing change.
  - **Be Safe!** Keep the PN solution refrigerated until 1 hour before use; do not give cold. Do not hasten warming by placing in a microwave oven or hot water bath.
  - **Be Safe!** IV tubing and equipment must be free of plasticizers (DEHP) when fat emulsion is to be infused.

Assessment
- Check the patient record for prescriber's orders for type and concentration of additives and rate of infusion.
- Check agency policy. Some agencies require tubing and filter change with every bottle or bag. The CDC recommends changing the PN set every 72 hours and a fat emulsion set at least every 24 hours.

- Assess:
  - Nutrition status and nutritional needs (e.g., daily weights, I&O, lab results).
  - Blood glucose level.
  - Patency of the IV site. If PN is being administered continuously by pump and the infusion is running and there is no leakage from the insertion, you can begin the first few steps of the procedure.
- **Be Safe!** You must confirm that proper catheter tip placement has been established before the initial PN administration.

Post-Procedure Reassessment

These are immediate post-procedure evaluations. An extensive description of ongoing monitoring is beyond the scope of this handbook.

- Assess VS, I&O, and weight.
- Observe that the solution is infusing at the prescribed rate.
- Assess patient's tolerance to the infusion (e.g., observe for pulmonary edema; check lab results).
- Observe for skin rashes, flushing, color changes, or other signs of allergic reactions; notify the primary provider.
- **Be Safe!** Monitor blood glucose and do not increase the infusion rate until glycemic control is established.

Key Points

- Perform preprocedure assessments.
- Position the patient supine.
- Examine the PN solution for leaks, cloudiness, and particles. If the solution contains lipids, also look for a brown layer, oil droplets, or oil on the surface. Have a coworker verify.
- Identify the patient, using two identifiers; have identification verified by a second staff member.
- Compare the bag to the patient's ID band and with the original prescription.
- Observe meticulous sterile technique in the appropriate steps of the procedure. During all steps, observe careful aseptic (clean) technique. Or follow agency policy.
- Attach the new administration set to the new bag. Use a filter.
- Prime the tubing (either now or after placing in the pump).
- **Be Safe!** PN solutions must be administered by infusion pump.
- Place the tubing in the infusion pump; set the rate.
- Clamp the catheter and the old administration set.

- Remove gloves, perform hand hygiene, and don clean or sterile gloves (per agency policy).
- Carefully identify the correct IV catheter and lumen for the PN (usually the largest one).
- Scrub all surfaces of the needleless connector and Luer-Lok threads with an antiseptic pad for at least 15 seconds.
- Aspirate or flush to determine patency of the IV line.
- **Be Safe!** If you meet resistance when flushing, do not flush forcibly. Try measures such as repositioning the patient and asking him to cough. If you still cannot flush, notify the primary provider.
- **Be Safe!** Trace the tubing back to the patient, attach the new infusion tubing to the designated PN lumen, and secure the Luer-Lok connection. Have the patient perform the Valsalva maneuver when connecting the tubing for the new infusion.
- Start the infusion.
- **Be Safe!** Set pump alarms; be sure they are working.
- Label the tubing.
- **Be Safe!** If the infusion rate falls behind or the pump gives occlusion alarms:
- Check that the pump is turned on.
- Try measures to relieve occlusion: aspirate the line and flush gently, reposition the patient and ask him to cough, roll the shoulder or raise the arm on the side the catheter is on.
- Change the filter if it is clogged.
- If these measures do not work, change the pump and have it checked in engineering.
- Do not attempt to catch up by increasing the rate.

Documentation

- A special form may be used for documenting PN administration.
- Record the bag number, date and time hung, volume, type of fluid, rate of delivery, and additives.
- Document pre- and postadministration assessment data, including:
- Complications and response to therapy.
- Patient's tolerance of procedure.
- Results of fingerstick blood glucose checks.
- Weight.
- I&O.
- Document the date and time of dressing or tubing change (if performed).
- If insulin is required, record the type, amount, and route/site administered.

Wilkinson Procedure 26-6. Administering Lipids

For steps to follow in all procedures, refer to the first page of this book, Universal Steps for All Procedures.

Equipment

- Intravenous lipid solution (not refrigerated).
- Special tubing (infusion set) for lipids.
  - If a filter is used, it must be a 1.2-micron filter.
  - Be Safe! Infusion set must be without plasticizers (DEHP) and should be labeled to that effect.
- Needleless cannula (if using a split-septum needleless connector that requires it).
- 70% isopropyl alcohol or CHG-containing pads.
- Procedure gloves.
- Time tape.
- Infusion pump.
- I&O record.

Assessment

- Check the patient record for:
  - Anemia.
  - Coagulation disorders.
  - Abnormal liver, pancreatic, or respiratory function.
- Be sure the prescriber is aware of these factors; they do not necessarily contraindicate giving the PN.
- Assess for:
  - Rash.
  - Eczema.
  - Dry, scaly skin.
  - Poor wound healing.
  - Sparse hair.
- Check a peripheral IV site for erythema, infiltration, and patency.
- Check a central venous access site for erythema or other signs of infection.
- Take baseline VS just before infusing the lipids. (Note: Not all guidelines require this action.)

Post-Procedure Reassessment
- If ordered, monitor serum lipids 4 hours after discontinuing the infusion.
- Monitor IV site for:
  - Patency.
  - Infection, inflammation, and infiltration.
- Monitor for:
  - Symptoms of fat emboli.
  - Allergic reactions.
  - Lipid intolerance.

Key Points
- Gather and prepare the equipment.
- Position the patient supine.
- Be certain lipids are not cold.
- Examine bottle for a layer of froth or separation into fat globules or layers.
- Label the bottle with patient's name, room number, date, time, rate, and stop/start times. Label tubing with date and time.
- Be Safe! Compare the lipids bottle to the patient's wrist band and the original prescription. Have a coworker verify.
- Use new tubing for each bottle of lipids.
- Be Safe! Carefully identify the correct IV line and port for the infusion. Trace the tubing from the bag back to the patient. If infusing simultaneously with PN, use a separate port below the PN filter.
- Take VS before infusing, then every 10 minutes for 30 minutes, and observe for side effects.
- Place the primed tubing in the pump, thoroughly scrub the catheter injection port or the Luer-Lok threads and hub with an antiseptic swab, attach the lipids tubing, and lock/secure the tubing connection.
- Begin the infusion slowly. If no reactions occur after 30 minutes, adjust to the prescribed rate.
- Complete the infusion within 20 hours.
- Be Smart! When lipids are infused with PN, the lipid infusion must be completed within 12 hours.
- When the infusion is finished, discard the bottle and IV administration set. They cannot be reused.

Documentation

- A special form may be used for documenting lipids and PN administration.
- Document:
  - Bottle number, date and time hung, volume, type of fluid, and rate of delivery.
  - Status of dressing, and date and time of dressing or tubing change (if performed).
  - Patient's tolerance of the procedure and any problems encountered.
  - Pre- and postadministration assessment data and blood tests, if any.
  - Condition of the IV site.
  - Weight.
  - I&O.

Wilkinson Procedure 37-4. Managing Gastrointestinal Suction

For steps to follow in all procedures, refer to the first page of this book, Universal Steps for All Procedures.

Note: This procedure assumes an NG or other enteric tube is already in place and that its correct placement has already been verified.

Equipment
Initial Equipment Setup
- Nonsterile procedure gloves.
- Suction source (either a portable machine or piped-in wall source).
- Suction container and tubing; stopcock.

When Emptying the Suction Container
- Clean nonsterile procedure gloves.
- Graduated container (not needed if suction canister is marked for measuring).
- Antiseptic wipes.

When Irrigating the NG Tubing
- Nonsterile procedure gloves.
- Irrigation set (basin and bulb syringe or catheter-tip syringe).
- Normal saline irrigant (unless another irrigant is prescribed).
- Linen-saver pads.

When Providing Comfort Measures
- Nonsterile procedure gloves.
- Emesis basin, cup, and water for mouth care.
- Water-soluble lubricant.
- Cotton-tipped applicators.
- Tissues or damp washcloth.

Assessment
- Determine that an NG tube has been inserted and placement verified by x-ray.
- Verify the prescriber's order for type of tube and whether it is to be placed to suction or a drainage bag; also verify the type of suction to be used (low, high, continuous, intermittent).
- Auscultate for bowel sounds.

- Also assess the patient's ability to cooperate with the procedure and understand explanations. This procedure assumes an NG tube is already in place, so assessments are ongoing.

Post-Procedure Reassessment and Maintenance
- Periodically assess placement of the tube by a combination of methods (i.e., by checking pH of aspirate, by listening over the stomach with a stethoscope while injecting air into the tube, and by reviewing radiographic reports).
- Monitor patency of the tube, effectiveness of the suction, and tube connections.
- Follow agency policy or the primary care provider's prescription for irrigation of the gastric tube.
- It is common to irrigate with 30 to 60 mL of normal saline every 4 to 6 hours.
- Monitor the color of the drainage (should be green to gold).
  - Be Safe! If there is blood in the drainage, notify the primary care provider.
- Be Smart! If the NG tube does not drain:
  - Check for kinks or blockage.
  - Check the suction apparatus; if the container is higher than the patient's abdomen, lower it.
  - If still not draining, irrigate the tube, if there is no contraindication.
  - If the tube is still not draining and the patient is uncomfortable, notify the primary care provider.
- Assess the patient's ability to move about in bed while attached to the suction source.
- Monitor patient comfort (e.g., sore throat); monitor gastric distention, vomiting, and abdominal pain. Auscultate for bowel sounds.
  - Be Smart! Turn off suction while auscultating.
- Examine skin and mucous membranes around the insertion site (e.g., nares, abdomen).
- For clients undergoing prolonged GI suction, observe for hyponatremia and hypokalemia (i.e., fatigue, lethargy, confusion, seizures, muscle weakness, paresthesia, and cardiac dysrhythmias).
  - Be Safe! Review lab results and report symptoms to the primary care provider.

Key Points
Initial Equipment Setup
■ Connect and secure the suction source, collection container, and drainage tubing.
■ Don nonsterile gloves.
■ Connect suction drainage tubing to NG tubing.
■ Secure the NG tube to the patient's nose and gown.
■ If available, connect a stopcock to the open end nearest the patient.
■ Turn on the suction source to the prescribed amount.
■■ Be Safe! If there is no order, use low suction.
■ Observe that drainage appears in the collection container.

Emptying the Suction Container
■ Don nonsterile gloves.
■ Turn off the suction; close the stopcock (or clamp the tubing).
■ Empty the suction container and measure the contents.
■ Empty and wash the graduated measuring container, if used.
■ Cleanse the suction container port and close the stopper; place the container back in the holder.
■ Turn on the suction source.
■ Observe for proper functioning and tubing patency.

Irrigating the NG Tubing
■ Prepare the irrigation set.
■ Place a linen-saver pad on the bed under the NG tube.
■ Don nonsterile gloves.
■ Check for NG tube placement by a combination of methods.
■ Fill the syringe with 30 to 50 mL of saline.
■ Turn off the stopcock or clamp the NG tube.
■ Disconnect the NG tube from drainage.
■ Drain the suction tubing and turn off the suction source.
■ Turn on the stopcock or unclamp the NG tube.
■ Slowly instill and withdraw irrigant into the NG tube until fluid flows freely. Take care to not instill into the air vent.
■ Be Safe! Do not force the solution into the tube.
■ Turn off the stopcock or reclamp the NG tube.
■ Reconnect the NG tube to the suction tube.
■ Turn on the stopcock or release the clamp.
■ Provide comfort measures.

Providing Comfort Measures
- Don nonsterile gloves.
- Provide mouth care.
- Remove nasal secretions with a tissue, damp cloth, or cotton-tipped applicator.
- Apply water-soluble lubricant to the inside of each nostril.
- Check that the tape or tube fixation device is secure.

Documentation
- Record all drainage as output on the I&O record.
- Record the time, type, and volume of irrigations and drainage returned. Note color, odor, and consistency of drainage.
- Document:
  - Patient's emotional and physical responses to intubation.
  - Any evidence of tube or equipment malfunction, epigastric pain, distention, or vomiting.

Urinary

Wilkinson Procedure 27-2A. Collecting a Clean-Catch Urine Specimen (Midstream Sampling)

✔️ For steps to follow in all procedures, refer to the first page of this book, Universal Steps for All Procedures.

Equipment
- Prepackaged collection kit.
  - If no kit is available: Sterile specimen container; antiseptic solution; sterile cotton balls or 2 in. × 2 in. gauze pads.
- Washcloth or towel.
- Mild soap and water.
- 2 pairs of clean procedure gloves.
- Specimen identification labels.
- Bedpan or bedside commode for an immobile patient.

Assessment
- Assess the patient's cognitive level to determine whether the patient will be able to follow instructions.
- Assess for:
  - Conditions that may impair the patient's ability to assume the necessary position.
  - Mobility status (to help determine where the specimen will be collected).
  - Ability to control urinary flow.

Post-Procedure Reassessment
- Assess:
  - Characteristics of the urine (e.g., color, odor, clarity, crystals, blood, mucus).
  - Any difficulties with urination (e.g., pain, burning, dribbling, difficulty beginning).

Key Points
- Don clean procedure gloves.
- Wash the perineum or the penis first with soap and water if soiled; otherwise, use an antiseptic towelette. (For women, wash from front to back; for men, use a circular motion from urethra outward.)

- Ask the patient to begin voiding. After the stream begins, collect a 30- to 60-mL specimen.
- **Be Safe!** Maintain sterility: Do not touch the inside of the container or the container lid.
- Place a lid on the container, label the container with the patient's name, the date, and the time of collection, and transport it to the lab in a timely manner.
- Follow agency policy on additional packaging. Many facilities require packaging the container in a specimen handling bag.

Documentation
- Record urine volume in the patient record, per agency protocol; include time and date the specimen was collected.
- Document characteristics of the urine: color, odor, particulate matter, blood, clarity, or other qualities.
- Document any difficulty with voiding, including pain or burning with urination, frequency, or difficulty starting the urine flow.

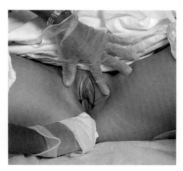

Cleansing the perineum using "clean to dirty" technique.

Wilkinson Procedure 27-2B. Obtaining a Sterile Urine Specimen From a Catheter

✔️ For steps to follow in all procedures, refer to the first page of this book, Universal Steps for All Procedures.

Equipment
■ Clean gloves.
■ Antiseptic swab.
■ Sterile specimen container with a lid.
■ Specimen identification label.
■ A 5- to 10-mL sterile syringe with a sterile 21- to 25-gauge needleless access device.

Assessment
■ Assess patency of the catheter (e.g., kinks).

Post-Procedure Reassessment
■ Observe for unusual characteristics of the urine (e.g., color, odor, clarity, crystals, blood, mucus).
■ Note any difficulties with urination (e.g., pain, burning, dribbling, difficulty beginning).

Key Points
■ Empty the drainage tube of urine.
■ **Be Smart!** If the client's urine is not flowing briskly, clamp the drainage tube below the level of the specimen port for 15 to 30 minutes to allow a fresh sample to collect.
■ Don clean gloves; swab the specimen port with an antiseptic swab.
■ Insert the needleless access device with a 20- or 30-mL syringe into the specimen port; aspirate the amount of urine you need.
■ Transfer the specimen into a sterile specimen container and cap it tightly.
■ Remove the clamp from the catheter and from the tubing of the urinary collection bag.
■ Label and package the specimen according to agency policy.
■ Transport the specimen to the lab. If immediate transport is not possible, refrigerate the sample.

■ **Be Safe!** Never disconnect the catheter from the drainage tube to obtain a sample. Interrupting the system creates a portal of entry for pathogens, thereby increasing the risk of contamination.

Documentation

■ Chart urine volume in the patient record, per agency protocol, including the time and date that the specimen was collected.

■ Record the characteristics of the urine: color, odor, particulate matter, blood, clarity, or other qualities; and any difficulty with voiding, including pain or burning with urination, frequency, or difficulty starting the urine flow.

■ You may also need to record urine output on the I&O record.

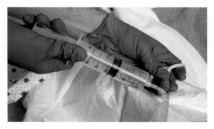

Obtaining a sterile urine specimen from a catheter.

Wilkinson Procedure 27-4B. Indwelling Urinary Catheterization

✔ For steps to follow in all procedures, refer to the first page of this book, Universal Steps for All Procedures.

Equipment
- Washcloth and towel; soap and water.
- At least 2 pairs of procedure gloves.
- Bath blanket.
- Procedure lamp or flashlight.
- 2% lidocaine gel (according to agency policy and patient need).
- Catheter insertion kit containing sterile gloves, antiseptic cleansing agent, forceps, cotton balls, sterile waterproof drapes, sterile lubricant, double-lumen or triple-lumen catheter with a balloon tip for inflation instead of a single-lumen rubber catheter.
- Syringe prefilled with sterile water.
- Tube holder, tape, or leg strap.
- Urine collection bag with drainage tubing attached (the tubing may also be attached to the catheter).

Assessment
- Assess the cognitive level to determine whether the patient will be able to follow instructions.
- Assess:
  - Conditions that may impair the patient's ability to assume the necessary position.
  - For signs and symptoms of bladder infection (e.g., elevated temperature, urinary frequency, dysuria).
  - Degree of bladder distention (to establish a baseline).
  - General size of the urinary meatus.
- Determine time of last voiding or last catheterization; allergy to iodine (if that is the antiseptic solution in the kit); and allergy to latex.
- Be Safe! Note conditions (e.g., enlarged prostate in men) that may make it difficult to pass the catheter.
- Be Smart! Assess the need for extra lighting.

Post-Procedure Reassessment
- Note:
    - Any difficulty with catheter insertion.
    - Characteristics of the urine obtained (e.g., amount, color, odor, presence of sediment or mucus).
    - Any bladder distention.
- Be Smart! Some facilities have a bladder-scanning device that will allow you to determine whether residual urine remains.
- Monitor to see that drainage is not obstructed and that the drainage bag is below the level of the bladder.

Key Points
- Be Smart! Allow adequate time for this procedure: Experienced nurses need at least 15 minutes. You will need more time if problems arise—and even more time if you are a novice.
- Be Smart! Take an extra pair of sterile gloves and an extra sterile catheter.
- Be sure to have good lighting.
- Work on the right side of the bed if you are right-handed; and on the left side if you are left-handed.
- Drape the patient for privacy.
- Perform perineal care before the procedure.
- Don sterile gloves and maintain sterile technique while manipulating the supplies in the kit and performing the procedure.
- Be Safe! Use a different solution for cleansing the perineum if the patient is allergic to iodine.
- Be Safe! For indwelling catheterization, pretesting the balloon by inflating it before insertion is not necessary, especially with silicone catheters, because the practice can cause the balloon to form cuffs. Cuffing can cause harm to the patient's urethra.
- Lubricate the catheter tip before insertion.
- Insert the catheter 5 to 7.5 cm (2 to 3 in.) for women, 17 to 22.5 cm (7 to 9 in.) for men, until urine flows—use the smallest size catheter possible.
- Be Smart! Once you have touched the patient's perineum with your nondominant hand, do not remove that hand from the patient.
- Drain the bladder; collect needed samples; measure urine; and connect the drainage bag.

Documentation

- Record:
  - Time and date of the procedure.
  - Size of catheter used.
  - Amount of urine obtained (on the I&O portion of the graphics sheet).
  - Color of urine.
  - Odor, presence of mucus and blood (in the nursing notes).
  - Patient's subjective statements.
  - Time a specimen was collected and sent to the lab.
- Some facilities require that you record the amount of saline used to inflate the balloon.

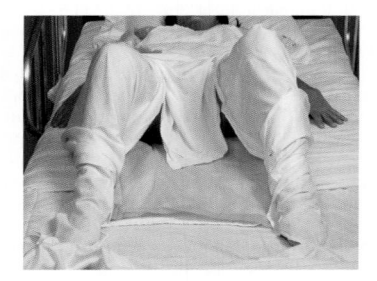

Draping a patient for privacy.

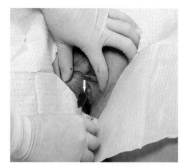

Cleansing the urinary meatus, through a fenestrated drape.

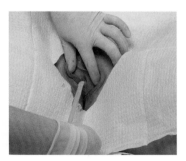

Inserting the urinary catheter.

Wilkinson Procedure 27-5. Applying an External (Condom) Catheter

✔️ For steps to follow in all procedures, refer to the first page of this book, Universal Steps for All Procedures.

Equipment
- Condom catheter.
- 2 pairs of clean procedure gloves.
- Washcloth and towel.
- Basin of soap and water.
- Bath blanket.
- Urine collection bag (e.g., bedside drainage bag or leg bag).
- Disposable tape measure.
- Skin prep (per agency policy).
- Scissors.
- Commercial leg strap.

Assessment
- Assess cognitive level to determine whether the patient will be able to follow instructions; and for conditions that may impair the patient's ability to assume the necessary position.
- Be Smart! Assess pattern of voiding to confirm that a condom catheter should be applied. Assess the skin along the shaft of the penis, the glans, and the meatus (for swelling or excoriation). Note whether and how much the penis is retracted toward the body.
- Be Safe! Assess for neuropathy that affects sensation in the penis and requires more frequent reassessment to prevent Impaired Skin Integrity.

Post-Procedure Reassessment
- Assess the penis for circulatory changes.
- Assess:
  - Position and patency of the drainage tubing.
  - Characteristics of the urine (e.g., amount, color, odor, bleeding).
  - Patient comfort.
  - Leakage of urine.

- **Be Safe!** Within 30 minutes after condom application, assess that urine flow is not obstructed; and that the penis is not swollen or discolored.

Key Points
- Clean and dry the penis before catheter application.
- When applying the condom, stabilize the penis with your nondominant hand.
- Leave a gap of 2.5 to 5 cm (1 to 2 in.) between the condom and the tip of the penis to prevent skin irritation.
- Use only the tape supplied in the application kit to secure the catheter.
- For condom catheters that contain adhesive material on the inside of the condom, grasp the penis and gently compress the condom onto the shaft.
- Be certain that the tubing from the end of the catheter to the drainage bag is free from kinks.

Documentation
- Chart date and time of application of the external catheter.
- Note unusual findings in your assessment of the penis.
- Document characteristics of urine (e.g., color, odor, consistency, blood).

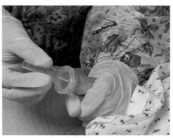

Unrolling the condom catheter.

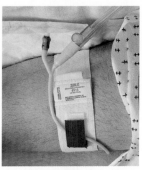

Securing the drainage tubing to the thigh using a commercial leg strap.

Wilkinson Procedure 27-6. Removing an Indwelling Catheter

✔ For steps to follow in all procedures, refer to the first page of this book, Universal Steps for All Procedures.

Equipment
- Syringe (5 to 30 mL, depending on balloon size).
- Towel or drape.
- Towel to use as a receptacle for the catheter.
- Hygiene supplies (washcloth, warm water, towel).

Assessment
- Assess:
  - Cognitive level to determine whether the patient will be able to follow instructions.
  - For conditions that may impair the patient's ability to assume the necessary position.
  - For bladder distention.
- Assess perineum and meatus (e.g., color, swelling, crusting, drainage, lesions).

Post-Procedure Reassessment
- Observe the condition of the meatus and the amount and characteristics of the urine; then monitor the next few voidings.
- Note the time of first voiding and amount voided, and observe the urine for color, amount, odor, and presence of blood.
- Compare voidings over the next 8 to 10 hours to the patient's intake.
- Monitor for bladder distention and signs and symptoms of infection.
- Be Smart! Place a collection container in the commode if the patient is ambulatory.

Key Points
- Use clean technique. Wash hands before and after removing the catheter. Wear clean procedure gloves.
- Be sure to remove the tape securing the catheter to the patient.
- Obtain a sterile specimen if needed.

- Deflate the balloon completely by aspirating the fluid.
- **Be Smart!** Check the balloon size on the valve port to verify that all fluid has been removed.
- **Be Safe!** If you cannot aspirate all the fluid, do not pull on the catheter.

Documentation

- Record:
- Date and time the catheter was removed.
- Amount of urine (on the I&O form).
- Characteristics of urine (e.g., color, odor, cloudiness, turbidity, or blood).
- Time the specimen was sent to the lab.
- Amount of fluid removed from balloon.
- Urine in drainage bag.
- Notification of first void.
- Unusual findings in your assessment of the perineum.
- How the patient tolerated the procedure.
- Patient teaching.

Wilkinson Procedure 27-7A. Intermittent Bladder/Catheter Irrigation

For steps to follow in all procedures, refer to the first page of this book, Universal Steps for All Procedures.

Equipment
Intermittent Irrigation Through a Three-Way Catheter
- Bag of sterile irrigation solution.
- Connecting tubing (to connect the bag to the irrigation port).
- IV pole.
- Antiseptic swabs.
- Bath blanket.

Intermittent Irrigation via the Specimen Port Using a Syringe
- Sterile container.
- Sterile 60-mL syringe with large-gauge needleless access device.
- 2 pairs of clean procedure gloves.

Assessment
- Assess:
  - Characteristics of the urine (e.g., amount, color, odor, presence of clots or mucus).
  - Presence and degree of bladder distention.
  - Discomfort.
  - Cognitive status (to know whether the patient can follow directions and not disrupt the sterile field during the procedure).
- Determine the amount and type of sterile solution to use.
- Determine how long the irrigant is to remain in the bladder.

Post-Procedure Reassessment
- Note:
  - Flow rate of irrigant and/or inability to instill irrigant into the catheter.
  - Characteristics of urine (e.g., presence of output, color, amount, clots, mucus).
  - Patient discomfort (e.g., pain, spasms).
  - Bladder distention accompanied by lack of urine outflow.

Key Points

- Establish a sterile field under the specimen removal port or the irrigation port on a three-way catheter.
- **Be Safe!** Because of the risk of infection, never disconnect the drainage tubing from the catheter.
- Use a sterile irrigation solution, warmed to room temperature.
- For intermittent irrigation using a three-way catheter, instill the irrigation solution slowly by gravity drain. The higher you hang the bag, the faster it will infuse in through the catheter.
- Repeat the process as necessary.

Documentation

- Chart:
  - Date and time of procedure, type of irrigant, and total volume infused.
  - Characteristics of the urine (e.g., color, odor, clarity, sediment, presence of clots or mucus).
  - Evidence of catheter patency (e.g., flow of urine, absence of distention).

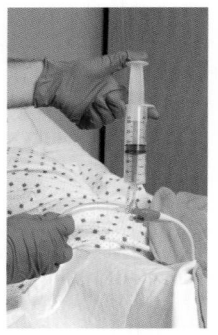

Holding the port above the bladder for irrigation.

Wilkinson Procedure 27-7B. Continuous Bladder/Catheter Irrigation

✔️ For steps to follow in all procedures, refer to the first page of this book, Universal Steps for All Procedures.

Equipment
- Three-way (or triple-lumen) indwelling catheter in place.
- Sterile irrigation solution at room temperature.
- Connecting tubing.
- Antiseptic swab.
- IV pole.
- Bath blanket.
- Measuring container.
- Pair of clean procedure gloves.

Assessment
- Assess:
  - Characteristics of the urine (e.g., amount, color, odor, presence of clots or mucus).
  - Bladder distention.
  - Patient discomfort.
  - Cognitive status.
- Check the chart for the amount and type of sterile solution to use and length of time the irrigant is to remain in the bladder.

Post-Procedure Reassessment
- Note:
  - Flow rate of irrigant and/or inability to instill irrigant into the catheter.
  - Characteristics of the urine (e.g., presence of output, color, amount, clots, mucus).
  - Patient report of discomfort (e.g., pain, spasms).
  - Bladder distention accompanied by lack of urine outflow.
- Monitor urine output.

Key Points
- Prepare the irrigation fluid and tubing:
  - Close the clamp on the connecting tubing.
  - Spike the tubing into the irrigation solution port, using aseptic technique.

- Invert the container, and hang it on the IV pole.
- Remove the protective cap from the distal end of the connecting tubing.
- Hold the end of the tubing over a sink or other receptacle.
- Open the roller clamp slowly, and allow the solution to fill the tubing completely.
- Recap the tubing.
- Perform hand hygiene and don clean procedure gloves.
- Place the patient supine and drape her so that only the connection port on the indwelling catheter is visible.
- **Be Smart!** Place a waterproof barrier drape under the irrigation port. If the irrigation kit comes with a sterile drape, use that.
- Pinch the tubing. Using aseptic technique, connect the end of the irrigation tubing to the side port of the catheter.
- Before beginning the flow of irrigation solution, empty any urine from the bedside drainage bag, and document the volume on the I&O record.
- Remove your gloves and wash your hands.
- Cover the patient, and return her to a position of comfort.
- Open the roller clamp on the tubing, and regulate the flow of the irrigation solution to meet the desired outcome for the irrigation.

Documentation

- Document:
- Date and time of procedure, type of irrigant, and the total volume infused.
- Characteristics of the urine (e.g., color, odor, clarity, sediment, presence of clots or mucus).
- Evidence of catheter patency (e.g., flow of urine, absence of distention).

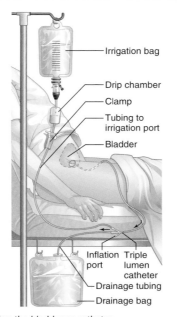

Irrigation bag

Drip chamber

Clamp

Tubing to
irrigation port

Bladder

Inflation Triple
port lumen
catheter

Drainage tubing

Drainage bag

Setup for irrigating the bladder or catheter.

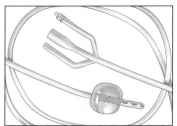

Triple-lumen irrigation catheter.

Wilkinson Procedure 28-2. Placing and Removing a Bedpan

✅ For steps to follow in all procedures, refer to the first page of this book, Universal Steps for All Procedures.

Equipment
- Bedpan.
- 2 pairs of clean gloves.
- Toilet tissue.
- 2 washcloths, towel, and basin.
- Waterproof pad.
- Bedpan cover.

Assessment
- Assess level of consciousness, ability to follow directions, and comfort level (especially note the presence of rectal or abdominal pain, hemorrhoids, or perianal irritation).
- Be Safe! Ask the primary provider to evaluate unexplained pain.
- Auscultate bowel sounds, and palpate for distention.
- Assess physical size and mobility; note whether the patient can sit up or lie flat when using a bedpan.
- Identify factors that necessitate the use of a fracture pan (e.g., fractured pelvis; total hip replacement; lower back surgery; casts, splints, or braces on lower limbs).
- Review the chart to determine the need to obtain a stool specimen.

Post-Procedure Reassessment
- Assess the amount and characteristics of urine and/or stool.
- Observe the skin on the perineum and buttocks for redness and breakdown.

Key Points
- Don clean procedure gloves.
- Be Smart! Help the patient to achieve a position on the bedpan that will be most helpful in facilitating urinary or bowel elimination. Use semi-Fowler's position whenever possible. Modify the position based on the patient's condition.

- **Be Smart!** Stabilize the bedpan when removing it.
- Provide toilet tissue, clean washcloths, and towels for the patient to perform personal hygiene when elimination is complete. Assist if the patient cannot perform these tasks independently.

Documentation

- Document the amount of urine voided if I&O are being recorded.
- Record any unusual characteristics of stool or urine in the nursing notes. If there are no unusual characteristics, you will probably document only in the graphic records.

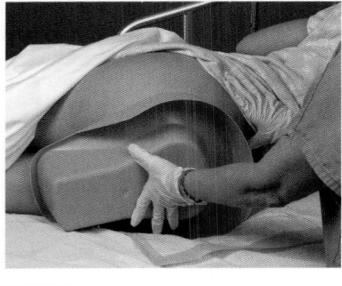

Placing a regular bedpan.

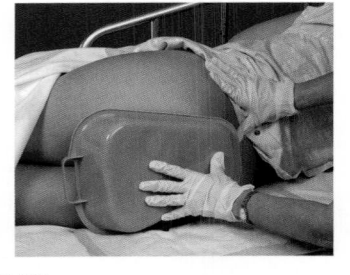

Placing a fracture pan.

Wilkinson Procedure 28-3A. Administering a Cleansing Enema

For steps to follow in all procedures, refer to the first page of this book, Universal Steps for All Procedures.

Equipment
- Washcloths, towels, disposable towelettes and/or toilet tissue.
- Bath blanket.
- Waterproof pad.
- Bedpan with cover or bedside commode, if needed.
- Water-soluble lubricant.
- Procedure gloves.
- IV pole.
- Enema administration container and solution, or prepackaged enema—depending on the type of enema ordered:
  - **Enema kit:** A package of supplies that includes a small plastic bucket or a 1-liter plastic bag with attached tubing, disposable toweling, lubricant, and castile soap.
  - **Prepackaged enema solution:** You may need to obtain a prepackaged enema from the pharmacy or central supply department.

Assessment
- Check for history of bowel disorders (e.g., diverticulitis, ulcerative colitis, recent bowel surgery, abdominal pain, abdominal distention, hemorrhoids) and for increased intracranial pressure, glaucoma, or recent rectal or prostate surgery.
- Be Smart! Review lab results (especially BUN, creatinine, and electrolytes). Hypertonic, hypotonic, and phosphate enemas have been linked to fluid and electrolyte changes.
- Inspect the abdomen for distention. Note the patient's last bowel movement, recent bowel movement pattern, and bowel sounds.
- Assess cognitive level and mobility status, degree of rectal sphincter control, and for presence of a fecal impaction.

Post-Procedure Reassessment
- Observe the amount, color, and consistency of the stool.
- Evaluate the patient's tolerance of the procedure (e.g., cramping, discomfort).

- Determine whether subsequent enema administration is required (e.g., a prescription for "enemas until clear").

Key Points
- Be Smart! Generously lubricate the rectal tube and insert it gently.
- Instill warm solution at a slow rate.
- Be sure patient is properly positioned.
- Instruct her to retain the solution for 3 to 15 minutes, depending on the type of enema.
- Assist the patient to a sitting or squatting position to promote defecation.
- Be Safe! Before leaving the bedside, implement fall prevention measures appropriate for your patient.
- Be Safe! Use nursing judgment to modify the procedure based on the patient's mobility and ability to follow instructions.

Documentation
- Document the type of enema given and, if applicable, the amount of the solution instilled.
- Document the patient's tolerance of the procedure and the characteristics and amount of the stool.
- If the prescription is to administer enemas until the returns are clear, document the color of the returned solution and the amount of stool seen.
- Be Smart! For prepackaged enemas, some facilities require documentation on the MAR.

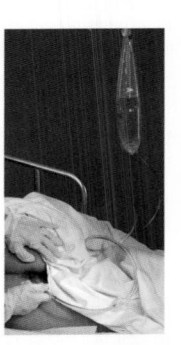

Start at the level of the patient's hips; then raise the container to 12 to 18 in. above hip level.

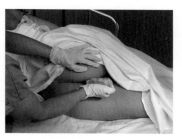

Administering a prepackaged enema.

Wilkinson Procedure 28-4. Removing Stool Digitally

For steps to follow in all procedures, refer to the first page of this book, Universal Steps for All Procedures.

Equipment
- 2 pairs of clean procedure gloves.
- Water-soluble lubricant (containing lidocaine, if agency policy permits).
- Bedpan and cover.
- Washcloth, soap, and towel or toilet tissue (or moistened towelettes).
- Basin of warm water.
- Bath blanket.
- Waterproof pad.

Assessment
- Assess:
  - Cognitive level and mobility status.
  - History of fecal impaction.
  - Time of last bowel movement.
  - Stool consistency.
  - Desire and ability to defecate.
  - Pain on defecation.
  - Pattern of bowel movements, diet, exercise, mobility status, and medications (e.g., iron supplements or narcotic analgesics).
  - Bowel sounds and abdominal distention.
- Be Safe! Assess the patient's baseline VS and history of heart disease. Be sure to monitor the patient's pulse before and during the procedure; be alert for bradycardia.
- Be Safe! Assess the patient's WBC count. If low, discuss this procedure with the primary care provider to evaluate the risks and benefits of the procedure.
- Be Smart! Determine whether the procedure will be accompanied by suppository insertion or enema administration.

Post-Procedure Reassessment
- Determine whether evacuation of the retained stool was complete. Perform a rectal exam to assess for presence of stool.
- Reassess VS, and compare the results to the initial assessment.
- Continue to monitor for 1 hour for bradycardia.

- Assess bowel sounds; palpate the abdomen for nontenderness and softness; ask the patient whether he feels relief from rectal pressure and abdominal discomfort.

Key Points
- **Be Smart!** Be aware that this procedure is both painful and embarrassing to your patient.
- **Be Safe!** Do not delegate this procedure to nursing assistive personnel.
- Trim and file your fingernails so they do not extend over the ends of your fingertips.
- **Be Smart!** You may wish to double-glove for this procedure.
- Lubricate your gloved finger generously.
- Use only one or two fingers, and remove stool in small pieces.
- Allow the patient periods of rest, and monitor for signs of vagal nerve stimulation.
- Teach the patient lifestyle changes necessary to prevent stool retention.

Documentation
- Document the bowel movement on the graphic record.
- Record the procedure and the patient's tolerance for the procedure, and any unusual characteristics of the stool (e.g., black or green color, blood, or mucus) in the nursing notes.
- Chart the pulse rate on the VS record.

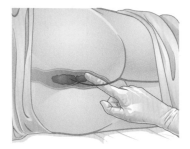

Gently rotate your finger around and into the mass.

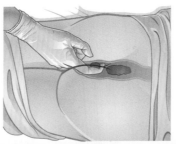

Break the stool into smaller pieces.

For steps to follow in all procedures, refer to the first page of this book, Universal Steps for All Procedures.

Equipment

- Skin care items per agency protocol (e.g., pH-balanced skin cleanser, skin prep, skin barrier wipe, adhesive remover, adhesive paste, and stoma paste if needed).
- Stoma measuring guide (or precut template).
- Scissors.
- Pen or pencil.
- 2 pairs of procedure gloves.
- Wash cloth, towel, basin with warm water.
- Toilet tissue.
- 4 in. × 4 in. gauze pad.
- Bedpan or container for effluent.
- Plastic bag for disposal of used pouch.
- Plastic bag for disposal of other contaminated articles.
- Waterproof pad.
- Ostomy deodorant.
- Hypoallergenic paper tape (optional) or ostomy belt.
- Bath blanket.
- Ostomy pouch:
  - One-piece pouch with the wafer attached, or a two-piece system with a separate wafer and pouch.
  - Clamp for pouches with an opening at the bottom (you do not need a new clamp each time).

Assessment

- Determine the changing schedule for the pouch and whether a new clamp is needed.
- Observe abdominal shape and incision, if present. Auscultate for bowel sounds.
- Assess the type of stoma (e.g., ileostomy, colostomy, urostomy), number of stomas, and location on the abdomen to determine the type of pouch to use.

■ Assess stoma color, shape, size, and/or length of protrusion or retraction; stoma construction (end, loop, double barrel); direction of stoma lumen; and discharge.

■ Be Smart! The stoma should be moist and red or pink. Alterations in color (purple, black, or blue) may indicate poor circulation and necrosis and should be reported to the primary provider.

■ Assess peristomal skin for redness, rash, irritation, or excoriation. Observe the existing skin barrier and pouch for leakage and length of time in place. You may have to remove the pouch to observe the stoma fully.

■ Be Smart! Notify the primary care provider or an ostomy specialist immediately if you note peristomal skin abnormalities.

■ Measure the stoma with each pouching system. Follow the manufacturer's directions and measuring guide for the size of ostomy pouch and the patient's stoma size.

Post-Procedure Reassessment

■ Observe:
  ■ Characteristics of stoma: color, size, presence of edema, and shape.
  ■ Presence of blisters, redness, or excoriation on peristomal skin.
  ■ Amount and characteristics of effluent: color, odor, consistency.
  ■ Whether the patient expressed a desire to participate in the task or demonstrated nonverbal cues that she is ready to learn about the task (e.g., looking at the stoma).
  ■ The patient's condition and self-care ability (consider vision, dexterity or mobility, and cognitive ability).

Key Points

■ Be Smart! Change the pouch every 3 to 5 days, as a general rule.

■ Empty the old pouch before removing it, if possible.

■ Remove the wafer or pouch, pulling down from the top with one hand while holding countertension with the other.

■ Assess the stoma and the peristomal skin area (e.g., for discoloration, swelling, redness, irritation, excoriation, bleeding).

■ Use a measuring guide to determine the size of the stoma.

■ Trace the size of the opening onto the back of the wafer, and cut the wafer opening about 2 to 3 mm (1/16 to ⅛ in.) larger.

■ Apply the new wafer with gentle pressure.

■ Some pouches come with the wafer attached, some without. These instructions assume that the wafer is attached.

Documentation

- Document:
  - Your assessment of the stoma and peristomal skin area.
  - Patient's tolerance of the procedure.
  - Type of appliance used, including the manufacturer and part number.
  - Use of any special ostomy skin care products.
  - Amount of liquid effluent (on the I&O portion of the graphics record).
  - Patient teaching and the degree to which the patient participated in the procedure.

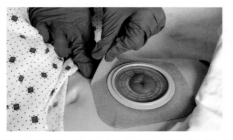

Apply adhesive remover with one hand as you press the skin away from the wafer with the other hand.

Wilkinson Procedure 28-7. Irrigating a Colostomy

✔️ For steps to follow in all procedures, refer to the first page of this book, Universal Steps for All Procedures.

Equipment
- Irrigation equipment:
  - One-piece system with a fluid container connected to tubing with cone; or two-piece system with a container separate from tubing and cone.
  - Irrigation sleeve; a sleeve without adhesive backing also requires a belt to hold it in place.
  - Clamp for a sleeve with an opening at the top.
  - Prescribed irrigating solution (usually 500 to 1,000 mL warm tap water, 100° to 105°F (37.8° to 40.6°C).
- IV pole or other equipment to hang the irrigation container.
- Chair.
- Water-soluble lubricant.
- Silicone-based adhesive remover.
- Skin cleansers and barriers as recommended by your agency.
- Toilet tissue.
- Washcloth, towel.
- Waterproof pad.
- 2 pairs of procedure gloves.
- Toilet facilities that include a flushable toilet and a hook or other device to hold the irrigation container (or bedpan or bedside commode for patients with impaired mobility).
- New ostomy appliance and skin barrier or stoma cap cover.
- Ostomy deodorant (optional).
- Plastic bag for disposal of the used pouch.

Assessment
- Assess cognitive level and mobility status.
- Assess the patient's ability to maintain a sitting position.
- Evaluate the defecation pattern, nature of stool, hydration status, placement of stoma, characterics of the stoma, abdominal distention, and nutritional pattern. Assess the type of ostomy.
  - Be Safe! Do not irrigate an ileostomy.

Post-Procedure Reassessment

- Observe:
  - Characteristics of the stool (color, amount, consistency).
  - Signs of bleeding from stoma or bowel.
  - Presence or absence of abdominal distention.
  - Patient's tolerance of procedure (e.g., cramps, fatigue).
  - Patient's ability to participate in the irrigation.

Key Points

- **Be Safe!** Consult with the ostomy nurse and/or physician to see if colostomy irrigation is appropriate for your patient.
- Determine the patient's normal bowel pattern before surgery.
- Prime the tubing before irrigation, using 500 to 1,000 mL, preferably 1,000 mL, of warm tap water.
- Hang the solution about 45 cm (18 in.) above the stoma height.
- **Be Smart!** Position the patient in front of or on the toilet or bedside commode. If the patient is immobile, place her in left side-lying (Sims') position, and use a bedpan.
- Prepare the new appliance before removing the existing one.
- Don procedure gloves.
- Examine the stoma and periostomal skin.
- Apply the irrigation sleeve.
- Lubricate the cone at the end of the tubing and insert it gently.
- Open the tubing clamp and let the solution flow slowly for about 10 to 15 minutes. Then clamp the tubing and remove the cone.
- Close the top of the irrigation sleeve with a clamp, have patient remain sitting, and allow approximately 30 minutes for evacuation.
- Remove the sleeve, and rinse, dry, and store it.
- Cleanse the stoma and peristomal skin with a warm washcloth.

Documentation

- Document:
  - Your assessment of the stoma and peristomal area.
  - The amount of irrigation solution used.
  - The date and time you performed the irrigation.
  - Characteristics of the stool returned in the irrigation fluid.
  - Patient teaching.

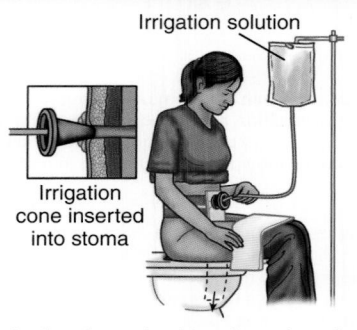

Irrigation solution

Irrigation
cone inserted
into stoma

The end of the irrigation sleeve should not hang down into the water.

Wilkinson Procedure 28-8A. Applying an External Fecal Collection System

For steps to follow in all procedures, refer to the first page of this book, Universal Steps for All Procedures.

Equipment
- pH-balanced soap and water or recommended skin cleanser.
- Skin protection wipes (e.g., peristomal wipes to protect skin and improve adherence).
- Self-adhesive fecal containment device.
- Procedure gloves.
- Linen-saver pad.
- Scissors.

Assessment
- Assess bowel patterns (fecal diversion is indicated when the patient is incontinent of liquid or semiliquid stools).
- Be Safe! Assess for contraindications to the use of an external fecal collection device; allergies/sensitivities to silicone or any of the materials in the device; impaired perirectal skin integrity.

Post-Procedure Reassessment
- Assess how well the patient tolerated the procedure.
- Note the color, consistency, and odor of stool.
- Monitor for abdominal distention and pain.
- Regularly assess that connections are secure and that the device is not leaking.
- Monitor the amount of stool in the collection bag.
  - Be Smart! Change the collection bag when it is about ⅔ full.

Key Points
- Select the fecal management system appropriate for the patient.
- Obtain assistance as needed.
- Place the patient side-lying.
- Don procedure gloves.
- Cleanse and dry perineal area; clip hair as needed.
- Spread the buttocks and apply the device; avoid gaps and creases.
- Connect the pouch to a drainage bag; hang lower than the patient.

Documentation

■ Record:

   ■ Date, time, and type of collection device used.
   ■ Assessment of the perineal skin.
   ■ Patient's tolerance of the procedure.
   ■ Characteristics and amount of stool in the collection bag (output).
   ■ Patient/family teaching.

Wilkinson Procedure 28-8B. Inserting an Indwelling Fecal Drainage Device

✔️ For steps to follow in all procedures, refer to the first page of this book, Universal Steps for All Procedures.

Equipment

- Fecal device kit: contains soft silicone catheter tube, a syringe, and a collection bag.
- Water-soluble lubricant.
- Approximately 100-mL container of tap water or saline (per manufacturer's directions).
- 500 mL of lukewarm irrigant (water or saline).
- 60-mL Luer-Lok syringe and a catheter-tip syringe (if not contained in the kit); protective skin-care dressing (e.g., Stomahesive).
- Tape, scissors, linen-saver pad.
- pH-balanced soap and water or recommended skin cleanser.
- Procedure gloves, mask, and goggles.
- Be Safe! Internal fecal catheters are not approved for children.

Assessment

- Assess recent bowel pattern. If no bowel movement for 2 or more days, the patient will likely need a bowel prep or enema before the procedure.
- Also check that a primary care provider has performed a digital rectal exam.
- Be Smart! The treatment plan may need to be changed if you discover the following:
  - Presence of any indwelling anal or rectal device (e.g., thermometer for continuous temperature monitoring).
  - Suppositories or enemas are a part of the current treatment plan. Collaborate with the primary provider, as needed.
- Be Safe! If the patient has a history of bowel disorders within the last 12 months (e.g., proctitis, recent rectal surgery; rectal injury or tumor; large and or inflamed hemorrhoids), contact the primary care provider immediately; an internal fecal catheter is contraindicated.

Post-Procedure Reassessment

■ Be Safe! Identify factors that increase the risk for bleeding, including anticoagulant and/or antiplatelet therapy and certain lab results (PT, PTT, platelets). These require careful patient monitoring.

■ Be Safe! Internal fecal devices are not intended for use longer than 29 days.

■ Be Safe! Monitor for rectal bleeding. It may indicate tissue necrosis, bowel perforation, or fistula formation; device must be removed.

Key Points

■ Obtain assistance as needed.

■ Don PPE.

■ Place the patient left side-lying and remove any indwelling device.

■ Cleanse and dry perineal area; clip hair as needed.

■ Prepare the device according to instructions (e.g., remove residual air from the balloon).

■ Connect the catheter to the collection bag. Clamp and hang the bag lower than the level of the patient.

■ Lubricate the balloon end of the catheter generously with water-soluble lubricant.

■ Spread buttocks and gently insert the balloon end of the catheter.

■ Inflate the retention cuff with water or saline.

■ Remove the syringe from the inflation port; gently tug the catheter.

■ Be Safe! If you used an introducer to insert the catheter, be sure to now completely aspirate the air from it.

■ If the device has anchoring straps, apply protective skin care dressing and tape one strap to each of the patient's buttocks.

■ Position the tubing, avoiding kinks; position the collection bag lower than patient.

Documentation

■ Chart:

■ Date, time, and type of collection device used.

■ Your assessment of the perineal skin.

■ Patient's tolerance of the procedure.

■ Characteristics and amount of stool in the collection bag (output).

■ Patient/family teaching.

Wilkinson Procedure 31-1A. Moving a Patient Up in Bed

☑ For steps to follow in all procedures, refer to the first page of this book, Universal Steps for All Procedures.

Equipment
- Nonlatex gloves, if you may be exposed to body fluids.
- Friction-reducing device, such as a transfer roller sheet or scoot sheet.
- Pull or lift (draw) sheet; pillows, as needed.

Assessment
- Assess:
  - Level of consciousness, ability to follow directions, and ability to assist with the move.
  - Any restrictions in movement or position.
  - Level of comfort, physical size, and assistive devices available.
  - Equipment in use, such as IV setups, pumps, or casts.

Post-Procedure Reassessment
- Assess:
  - Patient's comfort level.
  - Body position and alignment.
  - Skin for pressure areas.

Key Points
- Be Safe! Use a friction-reducing device to move the patient if the patient can assist with movement. Use a full body sling if the patient cannot assist.
- Remove the pillow. Have the patient flex her neck, fold her arms across her chest, and place her feet flat on bed.
- Position a nurse on either side of the patient.
- Be Smart! Use a wide base of support.
- Have the patient, on the count of 3, push off with her heels as you shift your weight forward.

Documentation

- Repositioning is not usually charted every time it is done; often it is recorded on a flowsheet.
- Document any problems with repositioning the patient or any areas of skin breakdown.
- You might also document turning as an intervention when charting to a specific problem. For example, for Impaired Skin Integrity, you might chart, "Position changed hourly."

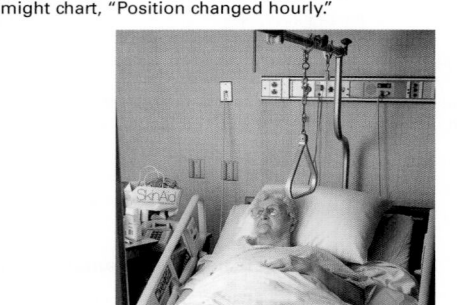

Move a patient up in bed using a trapeze.

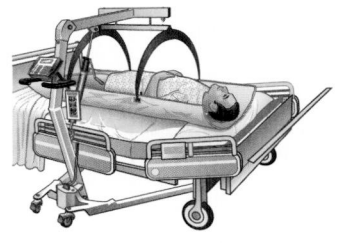

Move a patient up in bed using a mechanical device.

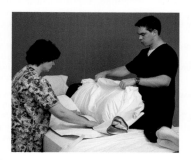

Use a drawsheet to turn the patient to one side of the bed.

Wilkinson Procedure 31-1C. Logrolling a Patient

✅ For steps to follow in all procedures, refer to the first page of this book, Universal Steps for All Procedures.

Equipment
- Nonlatex gloves, if you may be exposed to body fluids.
- Friction-reducing device, such as a transfer roller sheet or scoot sheet.
- Pull or lift (draw) sheet; pillows, as needed.

Assessment
- Assess:
  - Level of consciousness, ability to follow directions, and ability to assist with the move.
  - Any restrictions in movement or position.
  - Level of comfort.
  - Physical size of the patient.
  - Assistive devices available.
  - Presence of equipment such as IV setups, pumps, or casts.

Post-Procedure Reassessment
- Assess the patient's comfort level, body position and alignment, and skin for pressure areas.

Key Points
- Move the patient as a unit to the opposite side of the bed; raise the siderail on that side.
- Be Smart! Move to the side of the bed that the patient will be turning toward; lower the siderail.
- Be Safe! Each staff member evenly distributes his arms across the patient's length. One nurse is responsible for moving the head and neck as a unit.
- Shift your weight backward as you roll the patient toward you.

Documentation
- Repositioning is not usually charted every time it is done; often it is recorded on a flowsheet.
- Document in the nursing notes any problems with the procedure or any areas of skin breakdown.
- You might also document turning as an intervention when charting to a specific problem. For example, for Impaired Skin Integrity, you might chart, "Position changed hourly."

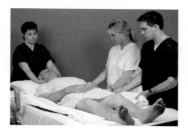

Logrolling a patient using a transfer roller sheet.

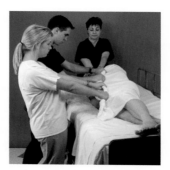

Logrolling a patient using proper body mechanics.

Wilkinson Procedure 31-2B. Dangling a Patient at the Side of the Bed

☑ For steps to follow in all procedures, refer to the first page of this book, Universal Steps for All Procedures.

Equipment
- Nonlatex gloves, if you may be exposed to body fluids.
- Transfer roller sheet or transfer board, if needed.
- Gait transfer belt.

Assessment
- Assess:
  - Level of consciousness, ability to follow directions, and ability to assist with the move.
  - The patient's physical size and your own ability to move him.
  - Restrictions in movement or position.
  - Patient's level of comfort; presence of equipment such as IV lines, drains, or catheters; possible side effects of medications (e.g., dizziness and sedation).
  - VS.
- Monitor for postural hypotension.
- Before transferring a patient to a chair, assess his tolerance of dangling.

Post-Procedure Reassessment
- Assess:
  - Level of patient participation in the transfer.
  - Comfort level during the transfer and in the new position.
  - Proper body position and alignment after position change.
  - VS for postural hypotension.

Key Points
- Place the patient supine, and raise the head of the bed to 90°.
- Be Safe! Apply a gait transfer belt, and put the bed in the low position with wheels locked.
- Stand facing the patient with a wide base of support. Place your foot closest to the head of the bed forward of the other foot.
- Position your hands on each side of the gait transfer belt.

- Rock onto your back foot as you move the patient into a sitting position; pivot to bring the patient's legs over the side of the bed.
- **Be Smart!** Stay with the patient as he dangles.

Documentation
- For nursing notes, document:
    - How much assistance was required.
    - Use of assistive devices.
    - Any problems with positioning the patient.
    - How long the patient was dangling.
    - How the patient tolerated the activity.

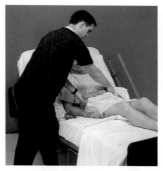

Using proper body mechanics for dangling a patient at the side of the bed.

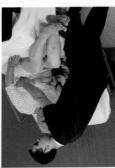

Pivoting the patient's legs to a dangle position.

Wilkinson Procedure 31-2C. Transferring a Patient From Bed to Chair

For steps to follow in all procedures, refer to the first page of this book, Universal Steps for All Procedures.

Equipment
- Nonlatex gloves, if you may be exposed to body fluids.
- Transfer roller sheet.
- Transfer board.
- Gait transfer belt.

Assessment
- Assess:
  - Level of consciousness, ability to follow directions, and ability to assist with the move.
  - Patient's physical size and your own ability to move her.
  - Restrictions in movement or position.
  - Patient's level of comfort.
  - Presence of equipment such as IV lines, drains, or catheters.
  - Possible side effects of medications (e.g., dizziness and sedation).
  - VS.
- Monitor for postural hypotension.
- Before transferring a patient to a chair, assess her tolerance of dangling.

Post-Procedure Reassessment
- Level of patient participation in the transfer.
- Comfort level during the transfer and in the new position.
- Proper body position and alignment after position change.
- VS for postural hypotension.

Key Points
- Be Safe! Instruct the patient to wear nonskid footwear (slippers or shoes).
- Place the bed in the low position, and lock the wheels.
- Assist the patient to dangle at the side of the bed.
- Brace your feet and knees against the patient. Bend your hips and knees, and hold onto the transfer belt.

- If two nurses are available to assist with the transfer, one nurse should be on each side of the patient.
- **Be Smart!** Instruct the patient to place her arms around you between your shoulders and waist. (The location depends on the height of the patient and the nurses.) Ask the patient to stand as you move to an upright position by straightening your legs and hips.
- Instruct the patient to pivot and turn with you toward the chair.
- Ask the patient to flex her hips and knees as she lowers herself to the chair. Guide her motion while maintaining a firm hold on her.
- **Be Safe!** If the chair is a wheelchair, lock the wheels.

Documentation

- Moving patients to a chair is a routine aspect of care and may not be documented.
- For nursing notes, document:
  - How much assistance was required.
  - Use of assistive devices.
  - Any problems with positioning the patient.
  - How long the patient was out of bed.
  - How the patient tolerated the activity.

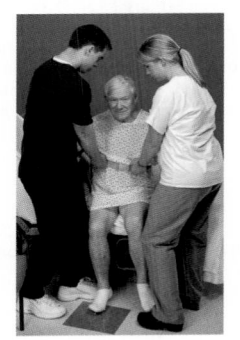

Transferring a patient from bed to chair by bracing feet and knees against the patient.

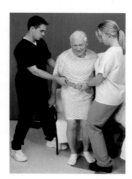

Transferring a patient from bed to chair using a transfer belt.

Wilkinson Procedure 31-3A. Assisting With Ambulation

✔ For steps to follow in all procedures, refer to the first page of this book, Universal Steps for All Procedures.

Equipment
■ Nonlatex gloves, if you may be exposed to body fluids.
■ Transfer belt.

Assessment
■ Assess:
  ■ Level of consciousness, ability to follow directions, and ability to assist with ambulation.
  ■ Physical size of the patient and your own ability to move the patient.
  ■ Factors that may increase the risk of falls (elderly, muscle strength, chronic disease, gait disturbance).
  ■ Any restrictions in movement or position.
  ■ Patient's level of comfort.
  ■ Presence of equipment such as IV lines, drains, or catheters.
  ■ Possible side effects of medications (e.g., dizziness and sedation).
  ■ VS (monitor for postural hypotension).

Post-Procedure Reassessment
■ Assess:
  ■ Level of patient participation in the transfer.
  ■ Patient's comfort with ambulation.
  ■ Posture and base of support.
  ■ VS for postural hypotension.

Key Points
■ Have the patient wear nonskid footwear.
■ Be Safe! Place the bed in low position, and lock the wheels.
■ Assist the patient to dangle at the side of the bed; assess the patient's tolerance before beginning ambulation.
■ If two nurses are available to assist with the transfer, one nurse should be on each side of the patient.
■ Be Safe! Brace your feet and knees against the patient. Bend your hips and knees, and hold onto the transfer belt. Pay attention to any known weakness.

- Instruct the patient to place her arms around you between your shoulders and waist (the location depends on the height of the patient and the nurses). Ask the patient to stand as you move to an upright position by straightening your legs and hips.
- Allow the patient to steady herself for a moment.
    - *One nurse:* Stand at the patient's side, placing both hands on the transfer belt. If the patient has weakness on one side, position yourself on the weaker side.
    - *Two nurses:* One nurse is on each side of the patient, grasping the transfer belt.
- Slowly guide the patient forward. Observe for signs of fatigue or dizziness.
- Be Safe! If the patient has an IV pole, allow the patient to hold onto the pole on the side where you are standing but not to use it for full support. Assist the patient to advance the pole as you ambulate together.

Documentation

- Record:
    - The amount of assistance required.
    - Any problems with ambulation.
    - The distance walked.

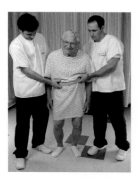

Stand at the patient's side, placing both hands on the transfer belt.

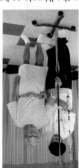

Assist the patient to advance the IV pole as he ambulates.

Wound Healing

Wilkinson Procedure 34-1. Obtaining a Wound Culture by Swab

✔️ For steps to follow in all procedures, refer to the first page of this book, Universal Steps for All Procedures.

Equipment
- 3 pairs of clean procedure gloves.
- Culturette tube.
- Sterile 4 in. × 4 in. gauze pad in an impermeable tray or separate 4 × 4 packs and an impermeable barrier.
- Sterile 0.9% (normal) saline solution for irrigation, warmed to body temperature.
- 35-mL syringe.
- 19-gauge angiocatheter.
- Gown and face shield.
- Emesis basin.
- Water-resistant disposable drapes.

Assessment
- If the wound is covered when you begin, you will make these assessments when you remove the soiled dressing *and* after cleansing the wound:
  - Assess for pain.
  - Determine whether the wound requires sterile, modified sterile, or clean technique.
  - Assess:
    - Amount and type of tissue present in the wound bed.
    - Type and amount of exudate.
    - Wound for odor.
    - Tissue surrounding the wound edge.

Post-Procedure Reassessment
- Assess patient's pain level and medicate according to prescriptions.
- Monitor lab reports for results of the swab culture.

Key Points

■ **Be Smart!** Position the patient for easy access to the wound and in a manner that will allow the irrigation solution to flow freely from the wound with the assistance of gravity.

■ **Be Safe!** Don protective equipment: gown, face shield, and clean procedure gloves.

■ Remove the soiled dressing and dispose of gloves and dressing.

■ Don clean gloves, and fill a 35-mL syringe with attached 19-gauge angiocatheter with 0.9% (normal) saline solution.

■ Holding the angiocatheter tip 2 cm (¾ to 1 in.) from the wound bed, gently irrigate the wound (superior to inferior).

■ Press the culture swab against an area of red granulating tissue, and rotate.

■ Reinsert the swab into the culturette tube, label the tube, and transport it to the lab.

Documentation

■ Chart:

■ Appearance and location of the wound and surrounding tissue, noting the type, consistency, and amount of exudate, and odor.

■ Patient's pain level before the culture. (If the patient was medicated for pain, document the drug and dose used, time given, and patient response.)

■ Method by which the wound was cleansed before the culture.

■ Description of the area where the culture was obtained.

■ Dressing reapplied to wound, if applicable.

■ Education provided to the patient.

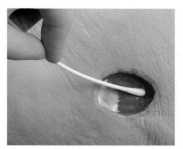

Collecting a wound culture by swab.

Wilkinson Procedure 34-3. Performing Sterile Wound Irrigation

✔️ For steps to follow in all procedures, refer to the first page of this book, Universal Steps for All Procedures.

Equipment

- Clean gloves.
- Sterile gloves.
- Gown and face shield.
- Water-resistant, disposable drapes.
- Tepid (body temperature) irrigation solution.
- Sterile gauze.
- Dressing supplies.
- Biohazard waste container.
- Sterile impermeable barrier.
- Sterile bowl.
- Sterile piston syringe or commercial irrigation kit (if irrigating with a syringe).
- If using an angiocatheter:
  - Sterile emesis basin.
  - 35-mL syringe.
  - 19-gauge angiocatheter (with needle removed).

Assessment

- If the wound is covered when you begin, you will make these assessments when you remove the soiled dressing *and* after cleansing the wound:
  - Amount and type of tissue present in the wound bed.
  - Whether the wound requires sterile, modified sterile, or clean technique for irrigation.
  - Assess the wound for:
    - Signs of infection (erythema, induration, amount and type of drainage).
    - Odor.
    - Periwound tissue.
    - Patient pain.

Post-Procedure Reassessment

- Determine whether the patient remains comfortable. If not, medicate according to prescriptions.
- Reassess the wound at regular intervals.

Key Points

- Administer pain medication 30 minutes before the procedure, if necessary.
- Position the patient for easy access to the wound and in a manner that will allow the irrigation solution to flow freely from the wound with the assistance of gravity.
- Be Safe! Don protective equipment: gown, face shield, and clean gloves.
- Remove the soiled dressing, and dispose of gloves.
- Set up a sterile field with a sterile irrigation kit or a 35-mL syringe and a 19-gauge angiocatheter (needle removed), dressing supplies, and irrigation solution.
- Wearing sterile gloves, fill either the syringe and angiocatheter or the piston-tip syringe with irrigation solution.
- Be Smart! Holding the syringe tip 2 cm (¾ to 1 in.) from the wound bed, gently irrigate the wound with a back-and-forth motion, moving from the superior aspect to the inferior aspect.
- Dry the tissue surrounding the wound with sterile gauze.
- Apply a new dressing as prescribed.
- Dispose of used equipment and soiled dressings in a biohazard waste container.
- Reposition the patient.

Documentation

- Document:
    - Appearance and location of the wound, size, tissue in wound base, periwound tissue, type and amount of exudate, and odor, after irrigation.
    - Patient's pain level.
- If the patient was medicated for pain, document the drug and dose used, time given, and patient response.
- Record:
    - Method by which the wound was cleansed.
    - Dressing reapplied to the wound, if applicable.
    - Education provided to the patient.

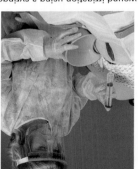

Performing a sterile wound irrigation using a syringe.

Wilkinson Procedure 34-6. Removing and Applying Wet-to-Damp Dressings

✔ For steps to follow in all procedures, refer to the first page of this book, Universal Steps for All Procedures.

Equipment

■ 3 pairs of clean nonsterile gloves.
■ Sterile solution or tap water for irrigation, warmed to body temperature when possible.
■ Water-resistant disposable drapes.
■ Sterile fine-mesh gauze in a tray for dressing.
■ Surgipad.
■ Tape or Montgomery straps.

Assessment

■ Assess:
  ■ Amount and type of tissue present in the wound bed.
  ■ Type and amount of exudate.
  ■ Wound odor.
  ■ Tissue surrounding the wound edge.
  ■ Patient pain.

Post-Procedure Reassessment

■ Verify that the patient experiences minimal discomfort with the procedure.
■ Note whether the patient verbalizes understanding of the procedure.

Key Points

■ Assess for pain, and medicate 30 minutes before procedure, if necessary.
■ Place the patient in a comfortable position that provides easy access to the wound.
■ Wearing clean gloves, remove the soiled dressing and discard it in a biohazard receptacle.
■ Be Safe! Change gloves and cleanse the wound with gauze moistened with sterile saline or tap water.
■ Assess the wound for location, appearance, odor, and drainage.
■ Don clean gloves and apply a single layer of moist, fine-mesh gauze to the wound. Be sure to place gauze in all depressions of the wound.
■ Apply a secondary moist layer over the first layer. Repeat this process until the wound is filled with moistened sterile gauze.

■ Cover the moistened gauze with a surgipad.
■ Be Smart! Secure the dressing with tape or Montgomery straps.

Documentation

■ Record:
  ■ Appearance and location of the wound, type and amount of exudate, and odor after cleansing.
  ■ Patient's pain level before the procedure.
  ■ Pain medication given including the dose, time, your name, and the patient's response.
  ■ Method of cleansing the wound.
  ■ Type of dressing applied to the wound.
  ■ Education provided to the patient.

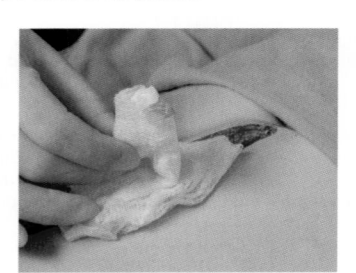

Removing a wet-to-damp dressing.

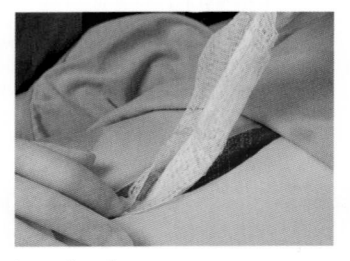

Packing a wet-to-damp dressing.

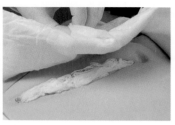

Covering a wet-to-damp dressing.

Wilkinson Procedure 34-7A. Applying a Negative Pressure Wound Therapy Device: Open-Pore Reticulated Polyurethane Foam (Vacuum-Assisted Closure)

✔ For steps to follow in all procedures, refer to the first page of this book, Universal Steps for All Procedures.

Equipment
- Suction unit (pump).
- Collection canister with connecting tubing.
- Dressing per manufacturer instructions.
- GranuFoam (black), white or silver foam dressing.
- TRAC pad.
- Semipermeable transparent adhesive dressing.
- Skin preparation product or sealant.
- Sterile 4 in. × 4 in. gauze pad.
- Clean procedure gloves.
- 2 pairs of sterile gloves (if using sterile technique).
- Sterile scissors (if using sterile technique).
- Waterproof pad.
- Bath blanket.
- Goggles or safety glasses, mask, and protective gown.
- 10- to 20-mL irrigation syringe.
- Normal saline for irrigation.
- Emesis basis.
- Biohazard bag for contaminated materials.

Assessment
- Assess wound type.
- Assess for:
  - Contraindication to use of an NPWT (e.g., nonenteric or unexplored fistulas).
  - Necrotic tissue with eschar.
  - Untreated osteomyelitis.
  - Malignancy in the wound or in exposed blood vessels.
  - Anastomotic sites, organs, or nerves.
- Assess for:
  - Active or prolonged bleeding.
  - Anticoagulant therapy or platelet aggregation inhibitors.
  - Presence of infected, damaged, irradiated, or sutured blood vessels.

- Assess the wound for:
  - Bone fragments or sharp edges, infection, or pain.
  - Size (length, width, and depth in centimeters).
  - Location and depth of undermining or tunneling.
  - Amount, character, and odor of drainage.
  - Type and percentage of tissue present in wound bed (granulation, slough, fibrin, necrotic).
  - Periwound condition (i.e., intact, denuded, erythema, induration, or maceration).
- Assess nutritional status.

Post-Procedure Reassessment
- Note the patient's response to the procedure.
- Continue to monitor wound healing and changes in periwound tissues.
- Monitor dressing every 2 hours to ensure it is firm and collapsed in the wound bed while therapy is on.
- Monitor the seal of the dressing, and pressure settings.
- Monitor for brisk or bright bleeding, evisceration or dehiscence, and symptoms of infection.

Key Points
- Administer an analgesic if needed.
- Select an appropriate dressing, per NPWT unit, to fill the entire wound cavity.
- Obtain a suction pump unit as prescribed.
- Prepare a sterile field for supplies.
- Don sterile gloves for new surgical wounds, or clean gloves for chronic wounds.
- Irrigate the wound.
- Apply appropriate dressing per NPWT unit.
- Cut the foam to fill the wound cavity.
- Be Safe! Do not place foam into blind/unexplored tunnels.
- Be Smart! Do not allow foam dressing to overlap onto healthy skin.
- Connect tubing attached to the dressing to the evacuation tubing going to the collection system.
- Be Safe! Position the tubing and connector away from bony prominences and skin creases.

- Ensure clamps are open on all tubing.
- Turn on the pump and set to prescribed settings.
- Listen for audible leaks and observe for dressing collapse or pruning.
- Change canister once a week or sooner if it fills.

Documentation

- Record:
  - Date and time of dressing change.
  - Wound assessment: location of the wound, size (length, width, diameter), undermining or tunneling, amount and character of drainage.
  - Odor.
  - Wound bed (including type and percentage of tissue seen, and peri-wound appearance).
  - Evaluation of therapy with evidence of healing.
  - Treatment selected (type of NPWT, type of gauze or foam, number of pieces placed in the wound).
  - Treatment settings (pressures, intermittent vs. continuous, or variable pressures).
  - Patient response to dressing change.

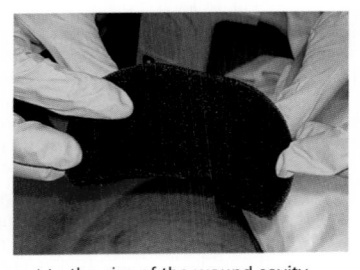

A foam dressing cut to the size of the wound cavity.

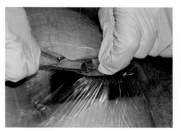

Pinching up a piece of the dressing to cut a hole.

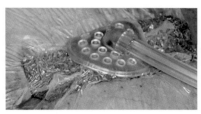

Applying the suction device for negative pressure wound therapy.

Wilkinson Procedure 34-9. Applying a Hydrating Dressing (Hydrocolloid or Hydrogel)

✔️ For steps to follow in all procedures, refer to the first page of this book, Universal Steps for All Procedures.

Equipment
- Clean nonsterile gloves.
- Hydrating dressing 3 to 4 cm (1.5 in.) larger than the wound.
- Moisture-proof bag.
- Obtain the following items only if needed:
  - Sterile normal saline solution for irrigation, warmed to body temperature.
  - Emesis basin.
  - Sterile gauze for cleansing.
  - Disposable clippers or scissors.
  - Skin prep.
  - Measuring device.
  - Tape.

Assessment
- Assess the area to determine whether a hydrating dressing is appropriate.
- Determine the size of the wound.

Post-Procedure Reassessment
- Note whether the dressing adheres comfortably to the skin.
- Ensure the patient verbalizes understanding of treatment.
- Inspect the dressing daily.
- Change it if it becomes dislodged, leaks, or wrinkles or if it develops an odor.
- Verify that a hydrocolloid dressing is still appropriate for the wound.

Key Points
- Place the patient in a comfortable position.
- Remove the soiled dressing, if necessary.
- Cleanse the wound, if necessary.
- Assess the wound, or other area where hydrocolloid dressing will be applied, for size, location, appearance, exudate, odor, and signs and symptoms of infection.

- **Be Smart!** Clip the hair around the wound if necessary.
- Apply the hydrating dressing.

Documentation
- Document:
    - Appearance and location of the wound, type and amount of exudate, and odor, after cleansing.
    - Wound measurements, if taken, and condition of surrounding skin.
    - Method of cleansing the wound and surrounding skin.
    - Type of dressing applied to the wound.
    - Use of skin prep.
    - Education provided to the patient.
- Assess the patient's pain level before the procedure.
- If the patient was medicated for pain, document the drug and dose used, time given, and patient response.

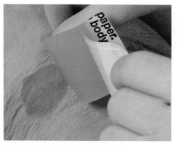

Removing the back of the hydrocolloid dressing.

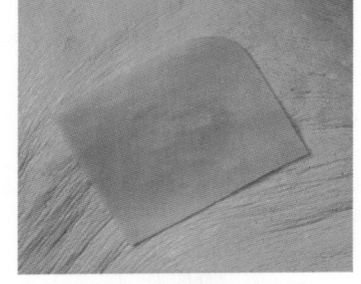

A hydrocolloid dressing after application to the skin.

Wilkinson Procedure 34-13. Removing Sutures and Staples

For steps to follow in all procedures, refer to the first page of this book, Universal Steps for All Procedures.

Equipment
- Nonsterile procedure gloves.
- Suture removal kit or sterile scissors and forceps.
- Staple remover.
- Gauze.

Assessment
- Assess staples to ensure none have rotated or turned instead of lying flat along the incision.

Post-Procedure Reassessment
- Note whether the incision is well approximated after the procedure.
- Ensure that the patient verbalized understanding of the treatment.
- Inspect the wound daily.

Key Points

Suture Removal
- Place the patient in a comfortable position.
- Remove the soiled dressing, if necessary.
- Use the forceps to pick up one end of the suture. Slide the small scissors around the suture, and cut near the skin.
- With the forceps, gently pull the suture in the direction of the knotted side to remove it.

Staple Removal
- Position the staple remover so that the lower jaw is on the bottom.
- Place both tips of the lower jaw of the staple remover underneath the staple.
- Lift slightly on the staple, ensuring that it stays perpendicular to the skin.
- Gently squeeze the handles together and lift the staple straight up.
- Place the removed staples on a piece of gauze.
- Dispose of the removed staples in the sharps container.
- Apply dressing, if needed.

Documentation

■ Document:
  ■ Appearance and location of the wound, type and amount of exudates, and odor, if present.
  ■ Patient's level of pain before and after the procedure.
  ■ Method of cleansing the wound and surrounding skin, if performed.
  ■ Removal of staples or sutures.
  ■ Education provided to the patient.

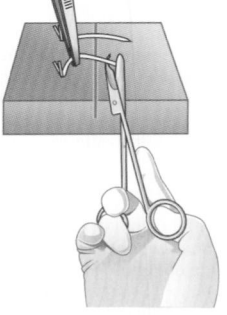

Removing interrupted sutures. Clipping the suture near the skin while using forceps to hold the knot.

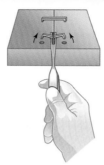

Removing a surgical staple.

Wilkinson Procedure 34-14. Shortening a Wound Drain

For steps to follow in all procedures, refer to the first page of this book, Universal Steps for All Procedures.

Equipment
- Nonsterile procedure gloves.
- Sterile gloves.
- Sterile scissors.
- 2 safety pins or other clips (sterile).
- Sterile gauze.

Assessment
- Inspect the site around the drain for skin excoriation, tenderness, erythema, warmth to the touch, and drainage from the wound.
- Assess characteristics of the drainage (color, volume, presence of blood, odor, or pus; and change in type or amount).
- Check the suction apparatus to be sure it is functioning properly.

Post-Procedure Reassessment
- Assess the skin around the drain after manipulating it. Note drain patency and be sure the drain is secure.
- Evaluate for complications occurring related to shortening procedure.

Key Points
- Using procedure gloves, remove the wound dressing. Discard in a moisture-proof biohazard container.
- Open sterile supplies and don sterile gloves.
- Be Smart! If the drain is tightly sutured in place, you might need to cut it with sterile scissors.
- Be Safe! Firmly grasp the full width of the drain at the level of the skin and pull it out by the prescribed amount (e.g., 6 mm [¼ in.]).
- Insert a sterile safety pin through the drain at the level of the skin. Hold the drain tightly, and insert the pin above your fingers.
- Using sterile scissors, cut the drain a little above the safety pin.

Documentation
- Record:
  - Amount and characteristics of the drainage.
  - Appearance of the wound.
  - Complications that occur (e.g., manipulation of tubing causes bleeding or drainage at the site).

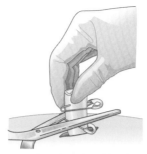

Cutting the drain between the safety pins, 1 in. above the skin.

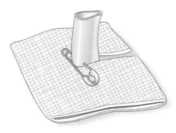

A precut gauze applied around the drain with safety pin at the base.

Wilkinson Procedure 34-15. Emptying a Closed-Wound Drainage System

✔️ For steps to follow in all procedures, refer to the first page of this book, Universal Steps for All Procedures.

Equipment
- Drainage container with graduated markings.
- Nonsterile procedure gloves.
- Disposal sink for biomaterial.
- Biohazard disposal receptacle.

Assessment
- Assess the appearance of the drainage tube site and sutures, if in place.
- Inspect for warmth, edema, redness, or pus where tubing penetrates the skin.
- Be sure the closed-wound drainage system is securely fastened at the connections and within the wound.
- Be Smart! Determine whether suction (electric, portable, or manual) is working properly.

Key Points
- Be Safe! Don PPE as needed, including nonsterile procedure gloves, gown, and eyewear.
- Properly dispose of contaminated items into designated biohazard waste receptacles.
- Measure drainage and report excess volume to the primary care provider.

Documentation
- Date and time the drainage system is emptied.
- Volume lost.
- Excess fluid loss.
- Appearance of drainage, including presence of blood or purulent material.

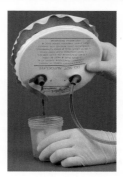

Opening the drainage port and emptying the fluid into a graduated container.

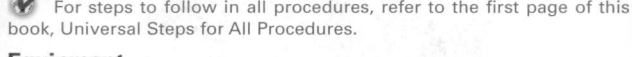

Oxygenation

Wilkinson Procedure 35-1A. Collecting an Expectorated Sputum Specimen

For steps to follow in all procedures, refer to the first page of this book, Universal Steps for All Procedures.

Equipment
- Sterile specimen container with lid.
- Procedure gloves.
- Glass of water.
- Emesis basin.
- Tissues.
- Linen-saver pad.
- Pillow (if abdominal or chest incision is present).
- Patient identification label.
- Completed laboratory requisition form.
- Small plastic bag (or agency-designated container) with a biohazard label for delivering the specimen to the laboratory.

Assessment
- Assess:
  - Comprehension of the procedure.
  - Ability to deep-breathe, cough, and expectorate.
  - Respiratory status (breath sounds; respiratory rate, depth, and pattern; skin and nailbed color; and tissue perfusion).
- Be Smart! You may need to delay sputum collection if the patient is in respiratory distress.

Post-Procedure Reassessment
- Evaluate the patient's respiratory status during and after the procedure.
- Examine the color, consistency, and odor of the sputum specimen.
- Evaluate the patient's understanding of the procedure and test results.
- Promptly report laboratory results to the primary care provider.

Key Points

- Use high- or semi-Fowler's position.
- Drape a linen-saver pad over the patient's chest.
- Instruct the patient to rinse his mouth and gargle with water.
- Caution the patient not to touch the inside of the sterile container or lid.
- Instruct the patient to breathe deeply for 3 or 4 breaths, hold his breath, and then cough and expectorate into the container.
- Repeat until an adequate sample is obtained (typically 5 to 10 mL).
- Label the specimen container with patient's name, test name, and collection date and time.
- Place the specimen in a plastic bag with a biohazard label. Follow agency policy.
- Send the specimen to the laboratory immediately.
  - If specimen transport is delayed, consult the lab; refrigeration may be required.

Documentation

- Record the date and time the specimen was collected, the method of collection, and the type of specimen ordered.
- Note the amount, color, consistency, and odor of the specimen.
- Document the patient's tolerance of the procedure.

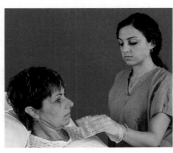

Ask the patient to rinse her mouth and gargle.

Wilkinson Procedure 35-2. Monitoring Pulse Oximetry (Arterial Oxygen Saturation)

For steps to follow in all procedures, refer to the first page of this book, Universal Steps for All Procedures.

Equipment
- Nail polish remover, if necessary.
- Oximeter.
- Oximeter probe sensor appropriate for patient age, size, weight, and for the desired location.

Assessment
- Check patient history for allergy to adhesive.
- Assess the patient's need for SaO_2 monitoring:
  - Risk factors, such as heart or pulmonary disease.
  - Low hemoglobin level.
  - Confusion, decreased level of consciousness.
  - Respiratory distress.
- Assess the patient's:
  - Respiratory status, including breath sounds.
  - Respiratory rate, depth, and pattern.
  - Tissue perfusion.
  - Skin and nailbed color.
- Determine the optimal location for the oximeter probe sensor (e.g., the fingertip, earlobe, forehead, or bridge of the nose).
- Check capillary refill and pulse at the pulse closest to the site.
- Assess for factors that may interfere with pulse oximetry measurement, such as hypotension, hypothermia, and tremors.
- Be Smart! To ensure accurate monitoring, choose a site that has adequate circulation, is free of artificial nails, and contains no moisture.
- Be Smart! Use a nasal sensor if peripheral circulation is compromised.

Post-Procedure Reassessment
- Evaluate the patient's understanding of the procedure and the obtained values.
- Compare pulse oximetry results with the patient's clinical presentation.

- Evaluate the effectiveness of therapy by comparing SaO_2 results before, during, and after treatment.
- Monitor skin integrity at the site every 4 hours if you are using an adhesive probe sensor or every 2 hours if you are using a clip-on probe sensor.

Key Points

- Choose a sensor that is appropriate for the patient's age, size, and weight and for the desired location.
- Cleanse and dry the site. Remove nail polish, as needed.
- Attach the probe sensor to the site. Photodetector and light-emitting diodes on the probe sensor should face each other.
- Connect the sensor probe to the oximeter, and turn it on.
- Check that the pulse rate on the oximeter corresponds with the patient's radial pulse.
- Read the SaO_2 measurement on the digital display when it reaches a constant value (usually in 10 to 30 seconds).
- Set and turn on the alarm limits for SaO_2 and pulse rate, according to the manufacturer's instructions, patient condition, and agency policy if continuous monitoring is necessary.
- **Be Smart!** Patients with underlying pulmonary disease may be accustomed to low oxygen saturation levels, so you may need to adjust the lower limit alarm.
- **Be Safe!** Rotate the site if monitoring is continuous.
- When monitoring is no longer needed, remove the probe sensor, and turn off the oximeter.

Documentation

- Most agencies use a flowsheet if frequent monitoring is necessary.
- Record the date and time of each pulse oximetry reading obtained; state whether readings are intermittent or continuous.
  - If readings are continuous, record alarm parameters.
- Chart the patient's vital signs and SaO_2 results, and indicate whether the patient is breathing room air or receiving oxygen therapy.
- If the patient is receiving oxygen therapy, note the oxygen concentration and the mode of delivery.
- Document acute decreases in SaO_2, any precipitating factors, treatment interventions, and the patient's response.

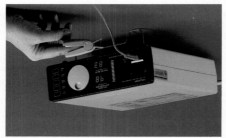

Pulse oximetry using a finger probe.

Wilkinson Procedure 35-5. Administering Oxygen

For steps to follow in all procedures, refer to the first page of this book, Universal Steps for All Procedures.

Equipment
- Oxygen source.
- Flow meter.
- Oxygen tubing.
- Nasal cannula, oxygen mask, or face tent.
- Prefilled humidification device.

Assessment
- Assess patient's understanding of oxygen therapy.
- Assess:
  - Respiratory status, including rate, depth, and rhythm.
  - Breath sounds.
  - Color.
  - Capillary refill and pulse oximetry results.
- Assess nares for patency (if a nasal cannula is being used) and behind the ears for signs of skin breakdown.

Post-Procedure Reassessment
- Assess respiratory rate, depth, and effort.
- Auscultate breath sounds before leaving the bedside, then monitor every 2 to 4 hours, and as indicated.
- Monitor pulse oximetry until respiratory status improves.
- Monitor ABG results if prescribed.
- Evaluate for skin breakdown, especially areas behind the ears, cheekbones, and under the chin—areas that are in contact with the oxygen delivery system.

Key Points
- Attach the flow meter to the oxygen source. Attach a humidifier to the flow meter, as needed.
- Assemble and apply the oxygen equipment according to the device prescribed (nasal cannula, face mask, or face tent).

- Attach the delivery device to the humidifier or the adapter, then put it on the patient:
  - *Nasal cannula:* Nose prongs should curve downward; loop the tubing around each ear; use the slide device to tighten the cannula under the chin.
  - *Face mask:* Secure the elastic band around the back of the head.
  - *Face tent:* Secure like face mask; be sure it fits under the chin.
- Turn on the oxygen using the flow meter, and adjust according to the prescribed flow rate.
- Double check that the oxygen equipment is set up correctly and functioning properly.
- Be Safe! Assess the patient's respiratory status before you leave the bedside.

Documentation

- Document:
  - Date, time, and reason oxygen therapy was initiated.
  - Type of oxygen delivery system used.
  - Amount of oxygen administered.
  - Patient's response to oxygen therapy.
- Record:
  - VS.
  - Pulse oximetry values.
  - Breath sounds.
  - Skin color.
  - Respiratory effort.

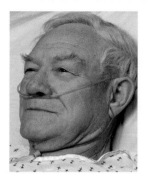

Nasal cannula.

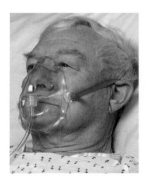

Face mask.

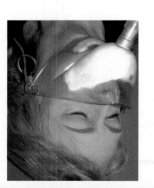

Face tent.

Wilkinson Procedure 35-6B. Performing Tracheostomy Care Using Modified Sterile Technique

For steps to follow in all procedures, refer to the first page of this book, Universal Steps for All Procedures.

Equipment
- Tracheostomy suction equipment.
- Tracheostomy care kit or the following sterile supplies:
  - Several cotton-tipped applicators, 2 basins, a brush, sterile 4 in. × 4 in. gauze pads, sterile precut tracheostomy dressing.
  - 2 pairs of procedure gloves.
- Disposable inner cannula that is the same size as the tracheostomy, if available.
- Normal saline solution or tap water if agency policy allows.
- Roll of twill tape or hook-and-loop fastener (Velcro) tracheostomy holder.
- Bandage scissors.
- Towel or linen-saver pad.
- Overbed table.
- Face shield.
- Protective gown.
- Mild soap and 2 clean washcloths.
- *For reusable inner cannula only:* hydrogen peroxide.

Assessment
- Assess respiratory status (i.e., rate, depth, and rhythm; breath sounds; color; and pulse oximetry results).
- Assess the tracheostomy site for drainage, redness, or swelling.
- Be Safe! Determine when the patient last ate. Schedule this procedure at least 3 hours after a meal to decrease risk of aspiration.

Post-Procedure Reassessment
- Assess the area around the stoma site for skin breakdown.
- Evaluate the patient's tolerance of the procedure and any signs of respiratory distress.

Key Points
- Position the patient in semi-Fowler's position.
- Don gown, eye protection, and gloves.

- Suction the tracheostomy.
- Remove soiled dressing; remove gloves; wash hands.
- Set up the sterile field and prepare equipment, keeping supplies sterile.
- Don clean procedure gloves.
- Remove the oxygen source if the patient is receiving oxygen, offer oxygen blow-by, and attach to the outer cannula. If that is not possible, clean and return the inner cannula before proceeding.
- Remove the inner cannula with your nondominant hand. If the cannula is disposable, discard it; if the cannula is reusable, clean it.
- Clean the stoma under the faceplate with the cotton-tipped applicators saturated with normal saline solution or tap water.
- Clean the top surface of the faceplate and the skin around it with the saline or water-soaked gauze pads, or with a washcloth and tap water. Dry the skin with dry sterile gauze.
- **Be Safe!** With the help of an assistant, remove soiled tracheostomy ties/stabilizer. If you must change ties without help, always place the new tape before cutting the soiled tape or holder.
- Ask the patient to flex his neck, and with an assistant stabilizing the tracheostomy tube, apply new tracheostomy ties.
- Insert a precut, sterile tracheostomy dressing under the faceplate and new ties.
- **Be Safe!** Use only sterile, precut dressing. Or open and refold a 4 in. × 4 in. gauze pad into a V shape. **Do not** cut 4 in. × 4 in. gauze, and do not use cotton-filled gauze squares.

Documentation

- Document date and time of the tracheostomy care.
- Note:
  - Color, amount, consistency, and odor of secretions.
  - Condition of the stoma and skin around the stoma site (presence of drainage, redness, or swelling).
- Record:
  - Respiratory status, including rate, depth, and pattern.
  - Skin color.
  - Breath sounds.
- Note the patient's tolerance of the procedure.
- Document any interventions that were needed.

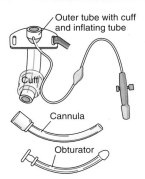

Disposable tracheostomy equipment.

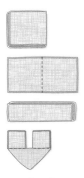

An unfolded and refolded gauze dressing.

Wilkinson Procedure 35-8. Performing Tracheostomy or Endotracheal Suctioning (Inline System)

For steps to follow in all procedures, refer to the first page of this book, Universal Steps for All Procedures.

Equipment
- *For the once-a-day steps:* procedure gloves; inline suction catheter.
- *When suctioning:* sterile normal saline.
- Be Smart! Inline suction is used only with a mechanical ventilator.
- Linen-saver pad.

Assessment
- Assess respiratory status (i.e., respiratory rate, depth, and rhythm; breath sounds; color; and pulse oximetry results).
- Assess for signs that indicate the need for suctioning:
  - Restlessness.
  - Cyanosis.
  - Labored respirations.
  - Decreased oxygen saturation.
  - Increased heart and respiratory rates.
  - Visible secretions in the airway.
  - Presence of adventitious breath sounds during auscultation.

Post-Procedure Reassessment
- Assess color, amount, and consistency of secretions.
- Evaluate the patient's tolerance of the procedure; note signs of respiratory distress during and after the procedure.
- Compare breath sounds, VS, and pulse oximetry before and after suctioning.

Key Points
Daily Procedure Steps
- Prepare the equipment.
- Open the inline suction catheter package, maintaining sterility.
- Remove the adapter on the ventilator tubing and attach the suction catheter equipment to the ventilator tubing.
- Reconnect the adapter on the ventilator tubing.
- Attach the other end of the inline catheter to the connection tubing going to suction.

Suction Procedure Steps

- Assist the patient to semi-Fowler's position unless contraindicated.
- Don clean gloves and place a linen-saver pad on the patient's chest.
- Unlock the suction control port.
- Adjust suction regulator according to guidelines or agency policy.
- Hyperoxygenate the patient according to agency policy.
- Unlock the inline catheter; with your dominant hand, insert the suction catheter gently, with suction off. Ask the patient to take slow, deep breaths if she can cooperate.
    - **Be Safe!** Do not apply suction as you enter or advance into the airway.
    - **Be Safe!** Advance the suction catheter gently, aiming downward, no further than the carina tracheae (premeasure). Do not force the catheter.
- Apply continuous suction as you withdraw the catheter, but for no longer than 15 seconds.
- Avoid saline lavage during suctioning.
- **Be Safe!** Repeat suctioning as needed, allowing intervals of at least 30 seconds between suctioning. Make sure to hyperoxygenate the patient between each pass.
- Withdraw the suction catheter completely into the sleeve, until you see the indicator line.
- Use normal saline to clear secretions from the catheter. Attach the prefilled, 10-mL container of saline to the saline port on the inline equipment; squeeze the container while applying suction.
- Lock the suction regulator port.
- Provide mouth care and reposition the patient.

Documentation

- Record:
    - Date, time, and reason for suctioning.
    - Size of suction catheter.
    - Amount, color, consistency, and odor of secretions.
    - Respiratory status before and after suctioning.
    - Patient's tolerance of the procedure.
    - Any complications as a result of the procedure, and interventions performed in response.

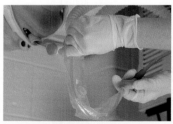

Insert into the airway by maneuvering the catheter within the sterile sleeve.

Wilkinson Procedure 35-10. Performing Upper Airway Suctioning

For steps to follow in all procedures, refer to the first page of this book, Universal Steps for All Procedures.

Equipment

- Portable or wall suction device with connection tubing and a collection canister.
- Linen-saver pad or towel.
- Yankauer device (can be used for oropharyngeal suction).
- Pour-bottle of sterile normal saline solution.
- Sterile basin or other container for fluids.
- Face shield or goggles and gown.
- Procedure gloves.
- Water-soluble lubricant for nasopharyngeal suctioning.
- Sputum trap, if a specimen is needed.
- Biohazard bag.
- Sterile suction catheter kit (12 to 18 Fr for adults, 8 to 10 Fr for children, and 5 to 8 Fr for infants).
- If a kit isn't available, collect the following: sterile suction catheter of the appropriate size, and a sterile container.
- If you plan to suction both the oropharynx and the nasopharynx, you need a separate sterile catheter for each.

Assessment

- Assess:
  - Respiratory status, including respiratory rate, depth, and rhythm.
  - Breath sounds.
  - Color.
  - Pulse oximetry results.
- Note signs that indicate the need for suctioning:
  - Restlessness.
  - Cyanosis.
  - Labored respirations.
  - Decreased oxygen saturation.
  - Increased heart and respiratory rates.
  - Visible secretions in the airway.
  - Presence of adventitious breath sounds during auscultation.

■ **Be Safe!** You must be certain the patient requires suctioning. Suctioning should be performed only when necessary to prevent unnecessary oxygen desaturation and tissue trauma.

Post-Procedure Reassessment
■ Assess the color, consistency, and amount of secretions.
■ Evaluate the patient's tolerance of the procedure.
■ Note whether there were signs of respiratory distress during the procedure.
■ Evaluate the effectiveness of the procedure by comparing breath sounds, VS, and pulse oximetry before and after the procedure.

Key Points
■ Position the patient in semi-Fowler's position.
  ■ *Oropharyngeal:* Patient's face turned toward you.
  ■ *Nasopharyngeal:* Neck hyperextended.
■ Adjust the suction regulator according to agency policy (typically 100 to 120 mm Hg for adults, 95 to 110 mm Hg for children, and 50 to 95 mm Hg for infants).
■ If using the nasal approach, open the water-soluble lubricant.
■ Don procedure gloves.
■ Using your dominant hand, attach the suction catheter to the connection tubing.
■ Approximate the depth the suction catheter should be inserted.
■ Remove the oxygen delivery device, if necessary.
■ If the oxygen saturation is less than 94%, or if patient is in distress, administer supplemental oxygen before, during, and after suctioning.
■ Lubricate and insert the suction catheter.
■ Gently advance the catheter the premeasured distance into the pharynx.
■ Engage the suction and apply it while you withdraw the catheter, using a continuous rotating motion.
■ Clear the catheter with sterile saline.
■ Lubricate the catheter, and repeat suctioning as needed, allowing 20-second intervals between suctioning.
■ **Be Smart!** Upper airway suctioning may be done via the oropharyngeal or nasopharyngeal route. However, nasal suction is usually required to improve oxygenation only in infants because most adult airway obstruction occurs in the mouth and oropharynx.
■ **Be Safe!** Vigorous nasal suction can induce epistaxis (nosebleed) and further complicate an already difficult airway.

Documentation

- Record:
  - Date, time, and reason you performed suctioning.
  - Suction technique you used.
  - Catheter size.
- Note:
  - Color, consistency, and odor of secretions.
  - Patient's respiratory status before and after the procedure.
  - Patient's tolerance of the procedure.
  - Any complications that occurred as a result of the procedure.
  - Resulting interventions.

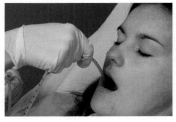

Oropharyngeal suctioning.

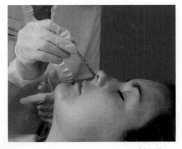

Nasopharyngeal suctioning.

Wilkinson Procedure 35-11. Caring for Patients Requiring Mechanical Ventilation

✔ For steps to follow in all procedures, refer to the first page of this book, Universal Steps for All Procedures.

Equipment
- 2 oxygen sources.
- Air source that provides 50 psi.
- Mechanical ventilator.
- Resuscitation bag with oxygen connection tubing.
- Humidification device.
- Ventilator tubing, connectors, and adaptors.
- Condensation collection device.
- Pulse oximetry device.
- Procedure gloves, protective gown, and eye covering.
- Sterile gloves and suction equipment, if you will perform suctioning.
- Suction equipment.
- Sterile water for the humidifier.
- Inline thermometer.

Assessment
- Review the health record to make sure that mechanical ventilation is included in the options outlined in the patient's advance directive.
- Assess the patient's understanding of mechanical ventilation therapy, if possible.
- Assess:
  - Respiratory status, including rate, depth, and rhythm.
  - Breath sounds.
  - Color.
  - Pulse oximetry results.
- Be Smart! Blood may be drawn for a baseline ABG analysis.

Post-Procedure Reassessment
- After mechanical ventilation is instituted, assess for chest expansion and auscultate bilateral breath sounds.
- Auscultate breath sounds every 2 to 4 hours, according to agency policy. Evaluate the patient's tolerance of mechanical ventilation.
- Verify adequate ventilation and that the patient is breathing in synchrony with the ventilator.

- ■ **Be Safe!** Check ABGs and respiratory status about 30 minutes after setup.
- ■ Monitor continuous pulse oximetry, capnography, and ABGs.
- ■ **Be Smart!** When monitoring VS, count spontaneous breaths as well as those delivered by the ventilator.

Key Points
Initial Ventilator Setup
- ■ Prepare the resuscitation bag; keep it at the bedside.
- ■ Respiratory therapists are responsible for setting up mechanical ventilation in most agencies. If you must assume the responsibility, refer to the manufacturer's instructions.
- ■ Plug in the ventilator and verify settings with the medical prescription.
- ■ **Be Safe!** Make sure the ventilator alarm limits are set appropriately.
- ■ Fill the humidifier with sterile distilled water.
- ■ Attach the ventilator tubing to the endotracheal tube or tracheostomy tube; secure the ventilator tubing.
- ■ Attach a capnography device, if available.
- ■ Prepare the inline suctioning equipment (see Procedure 35-8).

After the Initial Ventilator Setup
- ■ Wear gloves, protective eye covering, and gown.
- ■ Check respiratory status and ABGs again about 30 minutes after setup.
- ■ Be alert for changes in ventilator settings and the patient's compromised respiratory status.
- ■ Maintain the patient in a semirecumbent position (head of bed at 30° to 45°).
- ■ Check the ventilator tubing frequently for condensation.
  - ■ Drain the condensate into a collection device, or briefly disconnect the patient from the ventilator and empty the tubing into a waste receptacle, according to agency policy.
  - ■ **Be Safe!** Never drain the condensate into the humidifier.
- ■ Check ventilator and humidifier settings regularly.
- ■ Check the inline thermometer regularly.
- ■ Provide alternate form of communication (e.g., letter board, texting using a cell phone or keyboard).

- Reposition the patient regularly (every 1 to 2 hours), being careful not to pull on the ventilator tubing.
- Moisten the lips with a cool, damp cloth and water-based lubricant.
- Provide regular oral care: brush teeth twice a day with a soft tooth-brush, moisturize oral mucosa and lips every 2 to 4 hours, use mouthwash twice a day for adult patients.
  - Use a 0.12% CHG rinse twice a day for adult patients who have undergone cardiac surgery.
  - Be Smart! This regimen may help prevent VAP.
- Ensure that the call light is always within reach, and answer call light and ventilator alarms promptly.
- Monitor the tracheostomy tube for proper cuff inflation.
- Monitor for gastric distention.
- Give sedatives or antianxiety drugs as needed.

Documentation

- Note:
  - Date and time mechanical ventilation was initiated.
  - Type of ventilator and the prescribed settings used.
  - Patient's response to mechanical ventilation, including:
    - VS.
    - Breath sounds.
    - Ease of breathing.
    - Pulse oximetry.
    - I&O.
    - Skin color.
    - ABG and chest x-ray results.

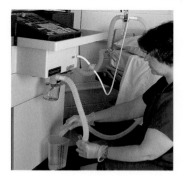

Drain tubing into a waste receptacle, never into the humidifier.

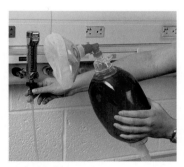

Preparing the resuscitation bag.

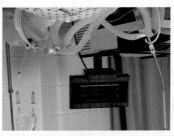

Verify ventilator settings.

Wilkinson Procedure 35-12. Setting up Disposable Chest Drainage Systems

✓ For steps to follow in all procedures, refer to the first page of this book, Universal Steps for All Procedures.

Equipment

- 2 disposable chest drainage units (CDU).
- Chest tube insertion kit (common tube size for adults is 36 Fr; kit should contain povidone-iodine, local anesthetic, syringe, needles, drapes, scalpel, suture).
- 5-in-1 or Y-connector for two chest tubes, if not contained in insertion kit.
- 2 rubber-tipped hemostats.
- Sterile gloves, masks, and sterile gowns.
- Sterile 4 in. × 4 in. gauze dressings.
- Sterile, precut drain dressings.
- Petroleum-based gauze dressings.
- Large drainage dressings (e.g., ABD).
- 2-in. silk tape.
- 1-in. silk tape or nylon banding system for securing tube connections.
- For a water-seal system, you also need sterile water.

Assessment

- Ensure that the patient has venous access.
- Assess:
  - VS.
  - Level of consciousness, orientation, responsiveness, anxiety, and restlessness.
  - Patient's knowledge of chest tube therapy.
  - Cardiac and respiratory status, including rate, depth, and rhythm.
  - Breath sounds.
  - Skin color.
  - Pulse oximetry.
  - ABG results.

Post-Procedure Reassessment

- Evaluate the patient's tolerance to the chest tube insertion.
- Determine whether the patient's respiratory status has changed after tube insertion.

- Auscultate breath sounds every 2 hours.
- Check type, color, and amount of chest drainage every 15 minutes for the first 2 hours, and then check as prescribed (at least every 4 hours).
- Assess for crepitus and drainage around the chest tube insertion site.
- Check the disposable chest drainage system for air leaks.
- Monitor I&O every 8 hours.
- Check laboratory values to evaluate blood loss and oxygenation.

Key Points

- Obtain and prepare the prescribed drainage system.
- Position the patient according to the indicated insertion site.
- Open the chest tube insertion tray and set up the sterile field.
- Don mask, gown, and sterile gloves and organize the supplies you will need for dressing the insertion site.
- As soon as the chest tube is inserted, attach it to the drainage system.
- Turn on the wall (or other) suction source (usually –80 mm H_2O).
- Set the prescribed CDU suction level (usually –20 cm H_2O).
- After the clinician sutures the chest tube in place, don a clean pair of sterile gloves.
- Be Safe! Using sterile technique, wrap petroleum gauze around the chest tube at the insertion site, and dress the site with two precut sterile drain dressings covered by a large drainage dressing (e.g., ABD).
- Be Safe! Apply an occlusive dressing over the insertion site (e.g., with 2-inch silk tape); cover the dressing completely. Date, time, and initial the dressing.
- Be Safe! Using the spiral taping technique, wrap 1-inch silk tape around the connections. Wrap from top to bottom and bottom to top. (Or use locking connections, if furnished with the CDU).
- With an 8-inch-long piece of 2-inch tape, secure the top end of the drainage tube to the chest tube dressing.
- Make sure the tubing lies with no kinks and no dependent areas, in a straight line to the CDU.
- Prepare the patient for a portable chest x-ray exam.
- Be Safe! Keep emergency supplies at the bedside in the event of tube dislodgement or system failure (2 rubber-tipped clamps, petroleum gauze dressing, and spare disposable CDU).
- Be Safe! Maintain the chest tube and drainage system by preventing kinks, ensuring patency of the air vent, and keeping the system below the level of the chest tube.
- Be Safe! Keep the head of the bed always elevated to at least 30°.

Documentation

- Document:
  - Assessment findings before, during, and after chest tube insertion (e.g., VS, breath sounds, cardiac status, pulse oximetry).
  - Date and time of the chest tube insertion.
  - Name of the clinician who performed the procedure.
  - Location of the insertion site, size of the chest tube, type of drainage system, and amount of suction applied, if any.
  - Any medications the patient received during the procedure.
  - Color and amount of drainage.
  - Patient's tolerance to the procedure.
  - Presence of subcutaneous emphysema or air leak, if any.
  - Complications and any interventions preformed as a result of the complications.
  - Chest x-ray findings.
- Record chest tube output on the I&O portion of the flowsheet (in most agencies).

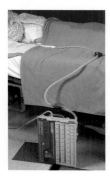

CDU set up and in place.

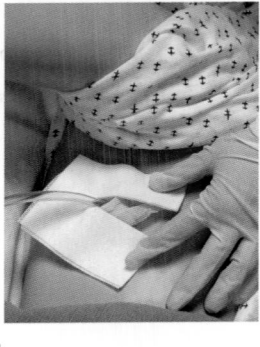

Precut drain dressing.

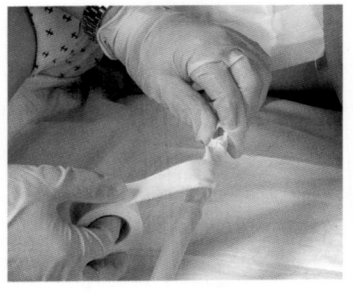

Spiral taping the connector.

Circulation

Wilkinson Procedure 35-3. Performing Cardiac Monitoring

For steps to follow in all procedures, refer to the first page of this book, Universal Steps for All Procedures.

Equipment
- Alcohol pads.
- Gauze pads.
- Washcloth.
- Shaving supplies or scissors, if necessary.
- Disposable electrodes.
- *For hardwire monitoring, add:* cardiac monitor; cable with lead wires; safety pin; 1-in. tape.
- *For telemetry, add:* transmitter with lead wires (with a new battery inserted before each use); pouch to carry transmitter.

Assessment
- Check for history of dysrhythmias.
- Assess cardiovascular status, including:
  - Heart sounds.
  - Pulse rate.
  - BP.
  - Check for the presence of pain.
- Be Smart! Assess skin integrity of the chest before applying electrodes.
  - Skin lesions contraindicate the application of leads to the affected area.

Post-Procedure Reassessment
- Evaluate changes in the patient's cardiac rhythm.
- Check skin integrity, and replace the electrodes at least every 24 hours.

Key Points
- Plug in the monitor and turn it on. Connect the cable with lead wires into the monitor.
- Identify electrode sites based on the monitoring system and the patient's anatomy.
- Gently rub the placement sites with a gauze pad until the skin reddens slightly.

- Use an alcohol pad to clean the areas for electrode placement; allow to dry.
- Connect lead wires to the electrodes.
- Be Smart! If the patient's chest is very hairy, shave small areas for the electrodes.
- Apply the electrodes, pressing firmly.
- Check the ECG tracing on the monitor. If necessary, adjust the gain to increase the waveform size.
- Be Safe! Set the upper and lower heart rate alarm limits and turn them on.
- Obtain a rhythm strip by pressing the "record" button.
- Be Smart! If you are not getting a good reading, recheck the leads, replace leads, or move leads if necessary.

Documentation

- Chart the date and time monitoring was instituted and the monitoring lead selected.
- Document a rhythm strip every 8 hours and with changes in the patient's condition according to agency policy.
- Label the rhythm strip (if the monitor does not label it for you) with the date, time, patient's name, and room number.
    - Indicate on the strip when symptoms and treatment interventions occurred.
- Document the patient's response to treatment.

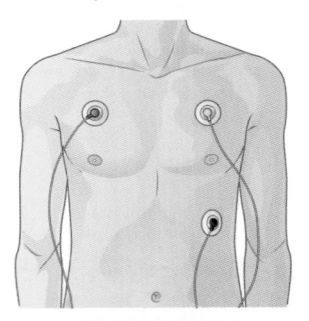

The monitoring system specifies lead placement.

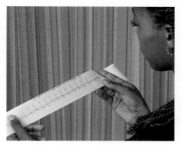

Evaluate the cardiac rhythm.

Wilkinson Procedure 37-1. Teaching a Patient to Deep-Breathe, Cough, Move in Bed, and Perform Leg Exercises

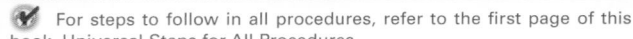 For steps to follow in all procedures, refer to the first page of this book, Universal Steps for All Procedures.

Equipment

For Teaching Deep Breathing and Coughing:
- Folded blanket or a pillow (if teaching will include splinting of a surgical incision site).
- Tissues.

For Moving in Bed:
- Small pillow or folded blanket.
- Pillows.

Assessment
- Assess cognitive level, level of consciousness, and pain level.
- Assess the patient's belief about the ability of the surgical incision to remain intact.
- Determine whether the surgical procedure or a physical disability will limit the patient's participation.
- Determine whether the surgical procedure may entail special exercises or equipment.
- Assess whether special equipment (e.g., braces, slings, or abductor wedges) may be needed when turning a patient in bed.
- Be Safe! For orthopedic surgeries, consult the surgeon before teaching the patient any leg exercises.
- Be Safe! Identify postoperative restrictions on movement (e.g., some spinal surgeries require the patient to logroll [move from head to toe as one unit]; some neurological procedures require limiting the amount of time the patient's head of bed is above 30°).
- Be Safe! Coughing and deep-breathing exercises are contraindicated for a patient who has had nasal, ophthalmic, or neurological surgery.

Post-Procedure Reassessment
- Make sure that the patient performs correctly a return demonstration of the procedures taught.

Key Points
- Assess the patient's readiness to learn.

Deep Breathing and Coughing
- Demonstrate how to splint a chest or abdominal incision.
- Use pillows to support the patient who is unable to maintain a side-lying position.
- Ensure that the patient is clear about the difference between coughing and merely clearing her throat.

Turning in Bed
- To turn to the left side: Start in supine position, bend the right leg, grasp the siderail with the right hand, and pull on the rail while pushing with the right foot. To turn to the right, repeat the process using the opposite limbs.

Leg Exercises:
- Teach the patient to alternately flex and extend her knees.
- Teach the patient to alternately dorsiflex and plantar flex her feet.
- Teach the patient to rotate her ankles in a complete circle.

Documentation
- Checklists and charts often have special areas in which to document patient teaching.
- Identify:
  - The person who completed the teaching.
  - The person to whom the procedures were taught.
  - What procedures were taught.
  - Whether the patient understood the teaching.
- Also include the name and type of any printed materials given.

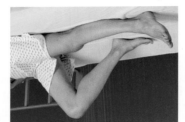

Performing leg exercises.

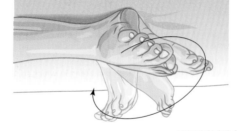

Performing ankle circles.

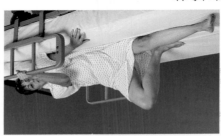

Turning to the left side.

Wilkinson Procedure 37-2. Applying Antiembolism Stockings

For steps to follow in all procedures, refer to the first page of this book, Universal Steps for All Procedures.

Equipment
- Measuring tape.
- Antiembolism stockings.
- Washcloth and towel (if needed to cleanse legs).
- Talcum powder (optional—check manufacturer's recommendations).

Assessment
- Assess:
  - Level of consciousness and cognitive ability.
  - Skin condition.
  - Be Safe! Assess for and symptoms of severe peripheral arterial disease, such as weak or absent pulses, discoloration or cyanosis, or gangrene. Antiembolism stockings may further impede arterial flow and should not be used in patients with any of these findings.
  - Be Safe! Assess the condition of the skin (lesions, dermatitis, or major edema, as evidenced by shiny, taut skin). Antiembolism stockings may irritate or worsen skin conditions and cause skin breakdown.

Post-Procedure Reassessment
- Evaluate patient comfort and ability to ambulate. Remeasure legs regularly to assess for edema and weight gain.
- Be Safe! Remove the stockings for 20 to 30 minutes every 8 to 12 hours and monitor skin condition. Check the stockings for wrinkles and/or rolling down at the top, especially when sitting.

Key Points
- Be Smart! Measure the patient's leg(s) to ensure that you select stockings of the correct size. Measure thigh and calf circumference at widest section.
  - *Thigh-high:* Measure distance from gluteal fold to base of the heel.
  - *Knee-high:* Measure distance from the middle of the knee joint to the base of the heel.

■ Be Smart! Place the patient supine for at least 15 minutes before stocking application. This prevents trapping of pooled venous blood.
■ Elevate the patient's legs for at least 15 minutes before applying stockings.
■ Cleanse legs and feet if necessary; dry well. Dust with powder if recommended by the manufacturer.
■ Insert your dominant hand to the heel, grasp heel and turn stocking inside out to the level of the heel with your other hand.
■ Insert patient's foot, toes pointed, into stocking. Gradually pull the remaining portion of the stocking up and over the leg.
  ■ Keep knee-high stockings 2.5 to 5 cm (1 to 2 in.) below the joint.
  ■ Be Safe! Do not apply thigh-high stockings if the thigh circumference is greater than 100 cm (25 in.).
■ Make sure the stocking is free of wrinkles and is not rolled at the top or bunched.
■ Be Smart! Launder stockings every 3 days.

Documentation
■ Document:
  ■ Leg measurements and size of the stockings used.
  ■ Time and date applied.
  ■ Condition of the skin, including any abnormalities.

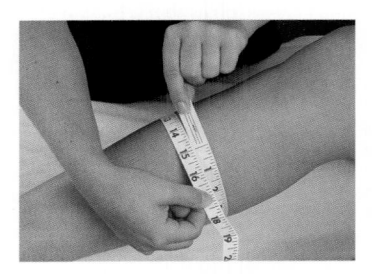

Measure the circumference at the widest part of the calf.

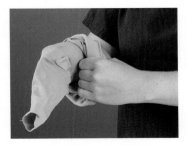

Grasp the heel with your hand inside the stocking.

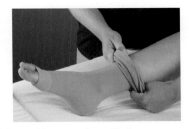

Gradually pull the stocking up and over the leg.

Wilkinson Procedure 37-3. Applying Sequential Compression Devices

✔️ For steps to follow in all procedures, refer to the first page of this book, Universal Steps for All Procedures.

Equipment
- Compression pump, motor, or machine.
- Connecting tubing, if applicable. (In some devices, the tubing is preconnected to the sleeves.)
- Compression sleeve (knee-high or thigh-high, depending on the prescription and the type of device).
- Elastic stockings (if prescribed).
- Washcloth and towel as needed to cleanse the lower extremities.
- Measuring tape.

Assessment
- Assess signs and symptoms of severe peripheral arterial disease (e.g., weak or absent pulses, discoloration, cyanosis, or gangrene).
- Assess the condition of the skin: note lesions, dermatitis, or major edema, as evidenced by shiny, taut skin.
- Be Safe! Assess cognitive level and level of consciousness. Patients with altered cognition may be at higher risk for falls related to the presence of the connecting tubing and attachment to the compression pump. Patients who are unconscious will not be able to report a device that is creating too much pressure.
- Be Smart! Increased compression of vessels by the sequential device may further impede arterial flow. If skin is overstretched by edema, the SCD may irritate or worsen skin conditions and cause skin breakdown.

Post-Procedure Reassessment
- Assess inflation and deflation of the sleeve to be sure the device is working.
- Monitor for kinking or pinching of the connecting tubing.
- Monitor circulation, sensation, and motion of the foot, including:
  - Skin color.
  - Pulses.
  - Temperature.
  - Capillary refill.
  - Motion and sensation.
  - Patient comfort.

- ■ Skin condition.
- ■ Signs and symptoms of deep vein thrombosis.
- ■ **Be Safe!** Remove the compression sleeves at intervals so that you can inspect skin and evaluate the adequacy of circulation. Note: If elastic stockings are being used in conjunction with SCD, follow the recommendations in Procedure 37-2.

Key Points

- ■ Determine whether elastic stockings are to be used concurrently with the SCD. If so, apply them (see Procedure 37-2).
- ■ Place the regulating pump for the sequential compression in a location that will ensure patient safety.
- ■ Place the patient in a supine position.
- ■ If you are using SCDS or PAS brand thigh-high compression sleeves, measure the thigh.
- ■ Place the lower extremity on the open sleeve, ensuring that the compression chambers are located over the correct anatomical structure (e.g., knee opening is at the level of the joint).
- ■ Leave one to two fingerbreadths between the sleeve and the extremity.
- ■ Set the regulating pump to the correct pressure, as prescribed.
- ■ **Be Safe!** Instruct the patient to call for assistance in disconnecting the tubing from the sleeve.

Documentation

- ■ Document the date and time you applied the device.
- ■ Note the type and size (if applicable) of the compression sleeve used.
- ■ Document the skin condition, including any abnormalities.

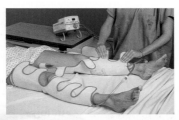

Sequential compression sleeves.

Abbreviations

ABG	Arterial blood gas
aPTT	Activated partial thromboplastin time
BP	Blood pressure
BUN	Blood urea nitrogen
CDC	Centers for Disease Control and Prevention
CDU	Chest drainage unit
CHG	Chlorhexidine gluconate
CVAD	Central venous access device
CVC	Central venous catheter
ECG	Electrocardiogram
FDA	Food and Drug Administration
GI	Gastrointestinal
HIPAA	Health Insurance Portability and Accountability Act
I & O	Intake and output
IM	Intramuscular
IV	Intravenous
MAR	Medication administration record
MDI	Metered-dose inhaler
NE	Nasoenteric
NG	Nasogastric
NPO	Nothing by mouth
NPWT	Negative pressure wound therapy
PEG	Percutaneous endoscopic gastrostomy
PICC	Peripherally inserted central catheter
PMI	Point of maximum impulse
PN	Parenteral nutrition
PPE	Personal protective equipment
PRN	As needed
PT	Prothrombin time
PTT	Partial thromboplastin time
ROM	Range of motion
SaO_2	Arterial oxygen saturation
SCD	Sequential compression device
TRAC	Therapeutic regulated accurate care
VAD	Vascular access device
VAP	Ventilator-associated pneumonia
VS	Vital signs
WBC	White blood cell(s)